I0023534

No Pain, Your Gain

How to Alleviate Back Pain and
Improve Your Workplace
Productivity

Lee Downer

No Pain, Your Gain
www.backcareworld.com

Copyright © 2017 by Lee Downer

All rights reserved. No portion of this book may be reproduced mechanically, electronically, or by any other means, including photocopying, without permission of the publisher or author except in the case of brief quotations embodied in critical articles and reviews. It is illegal to copy this book, post it to a website, or distribute it by any other means without permission from the publisher or author.

Limits of Liability and Disclaimer of Warranty
The author and publisher shall not be liable for your misuse of this material. This book is strictly for informational and educational purposes.

Warning – Disclaimer
The purpose of this book is to educate and entertain. The author and/or publisher do not guarantee that anyone following these techniques, suggestions, tips, ideas, or strategies will become successful. The author and/or publisher shall have neither liability nor responsibility to anyone with respect to any loss or damage caused, or alleged to be caused, directly or indirectly by the information contained in this book.

Not all exercise programs are suitable for everyone. Please consult with your doctor before beginning this or any other exercise program.

Publisher
10-10-10 Publishing
Markham, ON
Canada
Printed in the United States of America

ISBN: 978-1-77277-141-1

Contents

Dedication

*I dedicate this book to Roselda Ming (Mum)
and Veleta Anderson (nana) for taking care of me
when I couldn't take care of myself and, therefore,
saving my life on countless occasions.
Thank you both so very much (mothers);
I am forever in your debt.*

*With Lots of Love
Lee Downer (son)*

Testimonials

I have been a Dental Hygienist for over 25 years. A common hazard of my profession is chronic back, neck, and wrist pain. A close colleague of mine had to quit the profession due to severe back pain.

I have not experienced any of these problems, which I believe is the result of practicing CorYoga for many years. It has enabled me to be pain free and more agile, and to feel healthy. It also is helpful in relieving stress so you can handle life's challenges. I recommend CorYoga to everyone.

Connie Clark
Dental Hygienist

Out of about 20 teachers that I've tried in my life, most that taught in high-class places, I can confidently say that Lee is the best yoga teacher I've ever had! I was never too passionate about yoga and was about to quit it, until I met Lee. He has a unique combination of multiple characters that make him an outstanding teacher. First off, Lee is experienced, knowledgeable, and educated in the area that he teaches. He knows how to perfectly guide his students throughout class, instructing them step-by-step at a comfortable pace while both demonstrating, observing, and correcting his students. His voice is always calm, and his description of yoga positions are specific and clear. He always makes sure to bring a variety of the perfect music to every class that complements the environment perfectly. He knows when to make lighthearted jokes at the perfect moments, which are not distracting at all but rather put you at ease with him. I always walk out of his class feeling rejuvenated mentally and physically. If Lee would teach at the community every day, I would definitely take his classes daily. Thanks to Lee, I can confidently say that I am passionate about yoga. He has inspired me to integrate yoga into my life and grow on many levels because of it.

Miriam

I think that every workplace should make CorYoga back care classes available to its employees. It has increased my strength, flexibility, and circulation. Being able to simply concentrate on the moves and balance is a very relaxing process. CorYoga back care has also reduced my lower back pain that I sometimes get from sitting too long at my desk. I especially appreciate the 10 minutes of quiet time (Savasana – lying down, at the end); it helps to unscramble my thoughts and relax my mind. When I go back to work I am so much more focused and productive!

Stephanie F.
Fostering Sustainability
www.fosteringsustainability.ca

I have been doing CorYoga for almost 15 years now. I have acute back issues and, before I started with Lee, was seeing a chiropractor twice a week to deal with lower back pain. Over the 15 year period, my back pain has been significantly reduced due to Lee's CorYoga, to the extent where I now do not see my chiropractor twice a year!

My quality of life has improved tremendously, with little or no back pain, and I have Lee's CorYoga classes to thank for it.

Stephen A.
Accountant

I injured my back in an accident. After surgery, the rehab was extensive and lasted two years. I had physiotherapy, acupuncture, and chiro-practor treatment, and was on pain medication/ injections but always felt as if pain never left me.

It's been 5 years since I have been involved in midday CorYoga, twice per week, and because of CorYoga, I am able to live without back pain. In the last two years, I have travelled to the west coast of Canada, travelled to East and South Africa, and south and west of the USA.

I will be 70 shortly and, for me, breathing, relaxing, and getting energy are all the benefits I get from 1 hour of CorYoga. It helps me to keep my body and mind tuned up and to work on my muscles and joints that feel weak, before they become a problem.

Our life expectations are so demanding that we don't have time to relax and focus on our mind and body. CorYoga does this both.

We act when we have health or mental problems, but with CorYoga you eliminate that from happening. You have to dedicate some time for CorYoga; you will feel the difference.

Believe me, I know how my outlook has changed, and I am pain free.

Vic P.

Acknowledgements

Many amazing people and companies have graced my life and allowed me to grow and become who I am. First and foremost, I must give many thanks and praises to my three mothers, Roselda Ming (Mum), and Veleta Anderson. Without them, I most certainly would not have survived my early childhood. To my biological mother, Alva Aiken, who, with her amazing foresight, saved my life again by bringing me to Canada. Thank you Mothers, I am forever in your debt.

Among the many other amazing individuals and companies who have allowed me to present my "OYO Back Care for Office Workers" to their organizations are:

The MYCA of Canada: for initiating my growth to becoming the back care expert that I am by allowing me to teach their "Y's Way to a Healthy Back" program.
NBC Universal Studio (Grace dePasquale)
The Hudson Bay Company (North America's oldest company)
Nelson Thomson Canada (publishing company)

Thomson Carswell (Maureen Cooper)
Ontario Hospital Association (Isabella Wai)
North York General Hospital
Whitewater Golf and Country Club (Thunder Bay)
Financial Services Commission of Ontario (Provincial Government agency) (Donnette Vassell)
Ministry of Housing and Municipal Affairs (Provincial Government agency)
Human Resources Development Canada (HRDC) (Federal Government Agency) (Augustine Okan)
Canadian Management Centre (CMC) Conference exhibitor and presenter (Claudia Galban)
The Ontario Municipal Employees Retirement System (OMERS) (Joanna Fernandes)
The Toronto International Film Festival (Stefania Rigada)
Indas Canada (Chantal Cleroux)
The City of Toronto (Dorothea Pitt, Trecey Shand)
Extreme Fitness (Kamal Guirgis)
Fitness Connection (Christine Wong)
TD Bank
Herman Miller (Jane Heighten)
McMillan Binch LLP
AK Fitness Studio (Atif Khedri)
New Peaks: Robert Raymond Reopel and Michael Silvers

10-10-10 Publisher: Raymond Aaron
Alfe Grigg
Dr. Edward L. Demchuk: Chiropractic Doctor
Florence and the Machine
Bryan Adams
Black Eyed Peas
T-Pain Feat Tay Dizm
R. Kelly
Nancy Sinatra
Steve Winwood
Ronald William Eland
Neville Campbelle

Thank you all for helping to make me a better person and making this book possible.

With Love always,
Lee Downer

Foreword

I am extremely impressed with Lee Downer's back care strategies and his methods of healing back pain, as well as his extensive list of clientele. I highly recommend his book, *No Pain, Your Gain* to you, whether you are an office manager or a company executive.

No Pain, Your Gain contains proven techniques that will help you and your company's team to alleviate back pain and be the best you can be. As a result of having better health, you will take less sick days off for back pain, you will be more effective and efficient at work, and therefore you will be more productive. Alleviating and healing your back pain will result in improved profitability for your company.

If you are a company executive and would like to improve profitability through increased productivity, and at the same time take good care of your employees, then this book should be mandatory reading for you, and for all of your employees. Read No Pain, Your Gain now and learn how to care for your back!

Raymond Aaron
New York Times Bestselling Author

Chapter 1

The Visitor

My mother told me that ever since I was born I was never the kind of baby who would cry a lot. But on this one particular day, I started to cry for almost two days non-stop. Then, my mother's aunt, Cassie, came over and made me a special herbal bath in which she bathed me. After the bath, I stopped crying, and the crying spree went away. I was only 4 months old.

Why was I crying?

My paternal grandfather, David Downer, came to visit and took a look at me, his newborn grandson, but he came a little too close to me and frightened me. And that's why I started crying.

My grandfather, David Downer, had been dead for many years before I was born. He died when my father was just a little boy.

Why did I stop crying after the bath?

My mother's aunt, Cassie, was a spiritual healer and an herbalist; she washed away the residual effect of my dead grandfather's spirit that was still near me.

But is it really gone? Ummmm!!!!

It was early evening. The sun had already set and it was just starting to get dark when we heard the sound of Dun, the spiritual healer, coming. He was making strange grunting sounds that seemed to be coming from his throat. The sound was short, rhythmic, and steady. As he approached the house, we could see him dressed in long pants and short sleeve shirt, and his head was wrapped with a piece of cloth. He was hopping on one foot and was in a trance-like state. He had in his hand a strange piece of bush and was beating various parts of the ground with it. As he entered our yard, we knew why he came. He came to heal Mr. Lestan.

Mr. Lestan was sick. He became ill earlier that day and no one had told Dun that Mr. Lestan was sick. We lived about 3 miles away from where Mr. Dun lived and, without anyone telling him, he knew that Mr. Lestan was sick, so he came to heal him.

How did he know? GOK!

Spiritual healers know these things. I don't know how they know, but they do.

Have you ever noticed that if you were to bump your elbow, the first thing that you would do is immediately put your other hand on it?

Do you ever notice that?

The question is: why?

Why do you do that?

The answer is: INSTINCT.

You instinctively know that hands have healing power.

Think that through!

Assignment 1: Think of, and write down 5 things that you believe (we as humans) and know, instinctively.

Post your assignment on our website at www.back careworld.com

Mr. Lestan was my grandmother's second husband. He was not my father's father so we are not related by blood but, nevertheless, he was my step-grandfather. He got sick in the middle of the day, and by the evening he was in bed and couldn't move. Dun stayed and performed his ceremony well into the night. The ceremony involved singing and chanting strange non-understandable words and using a special herbal bush—beating it around various parts of the house inside and outside—so as to drive away the evil spirit that was causing my step grandfather to be sick. Within two days Mr. Lestan was better. Dun, the spiritual healer, was a maroon.

I am a maroon. We are maroons. The people of my village believe in witch doctors, voodoo, obeah, and spiritual healing. My people believe in jumbies, duppies, ghosts, and such. We are also herbalists; we believe that many illnesses can be cured with herbs. If you get sick, you would be taken to the spiritual healer. He would perform his ceremony with his herbs, singing and chanting, and within a few days you would be healed. Many people in my village were considered to be healers.

I am not sure if I believed in that part of my culture, but I was nevertheless one of them—a healer. I was not born to be a spiritual healer; I was born to heal back pain. I didn't know it and I didn't believe it, until recently.

This is my village:

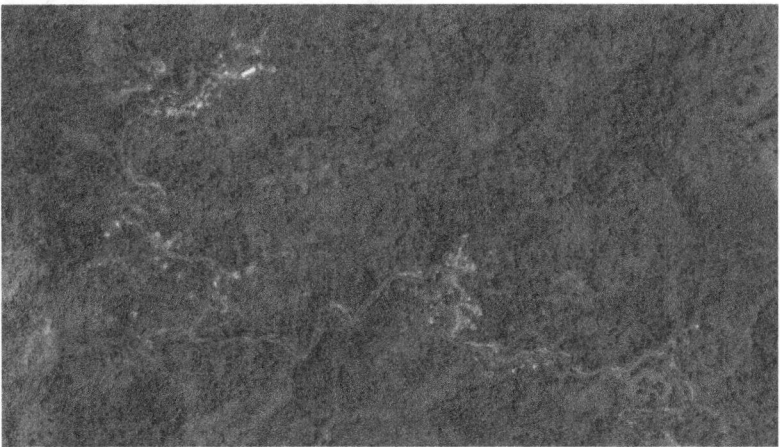

Fig. 1

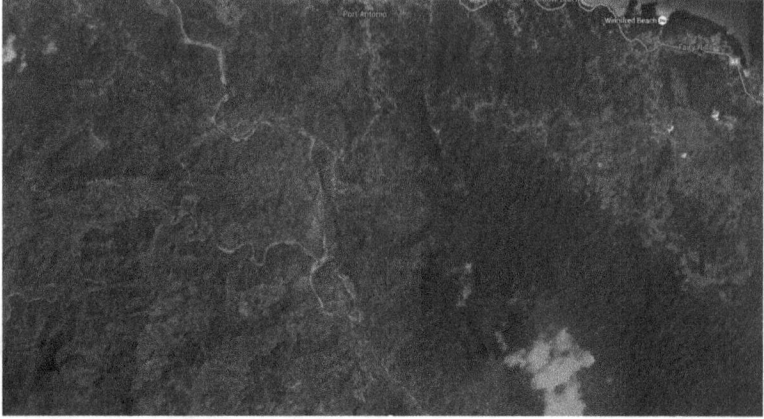

Fig. 2

The little grey spots to the left of the word google is my village. At the top of the picture in the centre, where it says Port Antonio, is civilization. This is how far up in the mountain I lived away from civilization.

I was born in a very small village in Portland, Jamaica (See the pictures, 1 and 2.). I was brought up by my Aunt Veleta and my grandmother, Mum. Her proper name was Roselda Ming. I spent the first 14 years of my life living with them, alternating between them.

The very first memories I have as a living human were not the happiest. I was always sick. I remember my Aunt Veleta putting me on her back and running with me to the healer man. I remember her giving me the strangest herbal tea to drink; when I refused to drink it, she would yell at me to "drink it." I remember her putting me against an apple tree and using a machete to chop above my head because it was believed that, by doing so, it would drive away evil spirits and heal my sickness—whatever that was, I haven't a clue. I just knew I was always sick. Every illness that went through my village (measles, chicken pox, mumps), I got them all, for me and for the rest of the kids in my village. When many of the other children didn't get sick, I did. I got my share of illnesses and their share as well. I was special—very special!! I was always a sick child. I was always being brought to the spiritual healer to be treated. It seemed to have worked since I am still here today.

My aunt has several nicknames for me, one of which was "Broken-Out." This is where my entire head, face included, became infested with little bumps which grew into bigger bumps, and then they broke-out into full-fledged sores; hence the name "Broken-Out." My head was one big sore. I couldn't comb my hair; my aunt just had to cut it very carefully because it was always very sore and painful.

Another nickname that my aunt called me was "Dead-An-Wake." She called me this because several times she was absolutely sure that I would not recover from one of my many illnesses. But she never gave up on me; and she was not my biological mother, only my father's sister. And so today, she and my grandmother are the ones I regard as Mother.

Then there was Paka Raka. This was the worst illness I have ever had, and this time I was living with my grandmother, Mum. Just as soon as I got over Broken-Out, I had Paka Raka. It started with little bumps all over my body that grew to become big bumps, and then became very itchy and broke out into sores all over my body this time. My body was full of little sores, literally from the bottom of my feet to the top of my head. I could not walk because when I stood, I stood on sores; when I lay down, I lay down on sores. I was a little boy. No child should have to go through this.

I was around 10 or 11 years old, and I still have very clear vivid memories of me standing in a wash pan while my grandmother, Mum, bathed me in a very special herbal bath that she prepared for me. The water was a bright, dark green colour from the herbs that she mushed up in the water. I can still remember myself feeling a little self-conscious of my grandmother washing my naked body and private parts, and thinking that I am a big grown boy. Not only should she not be looking at me and washing my private parts (I should be doing that for myself in private), we were in the middle of the yard for all to see. But I could not physically do anything for myself; I could not help myself because I was so very sick.

The fact that you are holding and reading this book that I have written with my own hands proved that I survived my sickly childhood. If it was not for the help of my grandmother and my Aunt Veleta, I most certainly would not have survived to tell about it, and nobody in Canada would ever have known me. I would not have survived because I would have been dead a long time ago.

I must also tell you that my grandmother, Mum, could not read or write. She was what you would consider by today's standards as illiterate, yet by using her alternative health and wellness knowledge and skills, she was able to save my life more than once.

Now why did I tell you that?

I tell you that, to tell you this. Do you need to be a medical doctor in order to treat some people and help them out of their pain? You decide for yourself, but all I can tell you is this: my so called illiterate grandmother who couldn't read or write was able to use her alternative remedies to save my ass over and over again, and I am eternally grateful to her for that. I can also tell you this: even though I don't even have a university degree, I have helped many people alleviate and eliminate their back pain, and am continuing to do so.

Thank you Mum. Thank you Aunt Veleta.

Remember this:

That which you were not good at, you will become expert at.

That which you consider to be a disadvantage, is your greatest advantage.

Consider this: why is it that people who suffer back pain know so much about the back pain?

It is because they took the time to study their situation so as to not have back pain; hence they become experts on back pain.

So, some of the things that I will suggest to you on how to alleviate your back pain, later on in this book, will be completely contrary to what some doctors will tell you. You will have to decide for yourself which to believe—a person with knowledge and no experience, or a person with 27 years of experience and some knowledge.

You decide.

Think about this: you would never hire someone who has no experience to work in your company, right? Then why would you take the word of some doctor (not all, just some) who has never experienced back pain, as if it is the word of God?

If that's food for thought, then eat up!

Consider this, which most people never consider: when a doctor tells you something about your back pain, have you ever asked them if they have ever suffered with your kind of back pain? How much experience do they have in suffering with your kind of back pain?

If I am a healer, then why make a healer start his life as a sick little boy? Well, when you have been very sick the way I have been, and then you recover and you get back your health, you can empathize with others. When someone says to you, "I am not feeling well," you don't just hear them; you feel what they are saying because you have been there already. You learn not to have a big ego because you remember how easily your health can be taken away. You learn to be humble. I have learned to be humble.

So, may I dare to say that I, Lee Downer, was born to be a healer?

You may be thinking, "What?"

You, "Dead-an-Wake?" You almost didn't even survive your childhood.

You, a healer? Hah hah hah hah!!!

I, too, had that very same thought. But then when I look back on my life and what I have done, I have come to realize that it was my destiny. I was destined to be a healer.

I have helped many people alleviate and eliminate their back pain because I have a good understanding of what is ailing them and how to fix it. Why? Because I have been very sick, and I got over it; and I have had back pain for 27 years and I have eliminated it, so I know how to heal most back pain.

That which you were not good at, you will become expert at.

That which you consider to be a disadvantage, is your greatest advantage.

And so I say to you, "How do you determine what is up if you have never experienced down? How do you know what is good if you have never experienced bad? How do you know good health if you have never been sick?"

So, take it from me, "Dead-An-Wake"—don't take chances with your health.

Remember:

He spent his health
To get his wealth,
With might in vain,
He spent his wealth
To get his health again

Race on over to chapter 2 to learn that there is no such thing as a bad thing.

Chapter 2

Nothing Bad Ever Happens

I left Jamaica and came to Canada in 1974. In 1975, I was at school playing floor hockey as part of my gym curriculum. During the game, the puck went into a corner of the floor, and I thought I heard the teacher blow the whistle, indicating a break in the game. As I casually walked over to get the puck, I was checked unexpectedly from the side. The sudden impact was so great that it threw one of my spinal discs (lumbar L4-L5 location) out of place. The spinal disc moved out of place and started pressing on my spinal nerve, causing pain, and in that same occurrence I almost broke my jaw. THIS WAS A BAD THING! Or so I thought. From that moment on, I had severe lower back pain. Of course, you can understand why; I had a bulging disc that was pressing on my spinal nerve while simultaneously causing inflammation, which compounded the problem.

I did not see a chiropractor until about two years later. I didn't know what a chiropractor was; I had never even heard of the word chiropractor, much less who they are or what they do. When I finally did see a chiropractor, two years later, he examined me and told me that I had a herniated disc, or a slipped disc or a bulging disc, and that one of my legs is slightly longer than the other as a result of me growing and not correcting the problem for the past two years. For the next 27 years, I lived with severe lower back pain.

But before I went to see the chiropractor, I first went to see my physician, and that was an interesting experience and diagnosis.

I remember the first time I went to my doctor about my back pain. He was a physician who had his office at the Pickering Town Centre. At that time, I had no idea what was going on with my back. All I knew was that I was having really bad back pain. I went to him and explained, to the best of my knowledge, the pain in my back. After he examined me, he couldn't find anything that was obviously physically wrong with me. He then asked me a very interesting question. He asked me, "Do you have a girlfriend?" I said, "No." He then said, "Go and get yourself a girlfriend; you need a girlfriend." I walked out of his office very confused. I had no idea what having sex had to do with the back pain that I was having. I thought that maybe there is some secret technique that will heal back pain. I was a teenager in high school and I wasn't sexually active yet. Let me also tell you that in high school I was a really nice guy. And subsequently, I never had a date throughout my entire high school career, and it wasn't for lack of trying. I was always asking pretty girls to go out on dates. But I always got the same standard answer. "Lee, you are a really nice guy, but I can't go out with you because if it doesn't work out, we wouldn't be friends anymore."

That ever happen to you? Uhhhhaaa!!!! Well, I got it all throughout high school and, subsequently, I never had a date in high school—not one.

Poor Lee!

A few months later, I went back to see my physician again about the same nagging back pain. After examining me again and not finding anything obvious wrong with me, he asked me again, "Have you got a girlfriend yet?" To which I answered, "No." He then said, "I told you, you need a girlfriend. Go and get yourself a girlfriend." I left his office and never went back to see that doctor, and I will never forget his name. (And no, I won't mention his name because I don't want his lawyer talking to my lawyer, if he is still alive.) I believe this man's ego was bigger than his career. He obviously didn't know what was wrong with my back and, instead of telling me he didn't know what was wrong with me, and sending me to see a chiropractor or maybe another physician that could help me, he decided to give me some cockamamie advice. Ever since then, I never went to see a male physician; I find female physicians to be more caring and more thoughtful, and more pleasing to my male eyes anyway. I realized that I may be doing myself some disservice, but this is what I have learned from experience and I therefore live by it.

Two years after graduating from college and getting a career as a draftsman, and after being a chiropractic patient for several years, my chiropractor said to me, "Lee, you know so much about backs, you should be a chiropractor." He said that if I would go back to university and get my bachelor degree in science, he would give me a personal endorsement to the Canadian Memorial Chiropractic College. He would see to it that I get in. He was on the Board of Directors at the Canadian Memorial Chiropractic College. It doesn't get any better; I was in good hands. Whaahooo!!!!

For the next two years, I repositioned myself, quit my job, and went back to university to study physical education and pure and applied science, in order to go to Chiropractic College. The only reason I went back to university was to become a chiropractor, which never happened.

In my first year at university, the YMCA hired me as a fitness consultant; there, I learned a lot and grew a lot.

Then, one day, the manager came up to me and said, "Lee, the yoga teacher did not show up to teach his class. Can you go upstairs and teach that class?" I said, "No, I don't know how to do it. I have never taught such a class before." She said to just do whatever I could because they really don't cancel classes; they just get others to sub the class. So, being a fitness guy studying Physical Education at the university and having a strong understanding of human physiology, I went upstairs and did the best I could. At that point, I had never heard the word yoga; I didn't even know how to spell the word yoga. Imagine that a university student doesn't know how to spell yoga. I know what you are thinking now. Don't call me that! Regardless of what you may think of me, I am still who I am, and I am still loving me.

But, from that day until this day, I have never stopped teaching yoga. Then, the YMCA sent me to various places to get formal training in various styles of yoga, all while I was still teaching my yoga class at the YMCA. As time went by, I got better. Then the Y assigned me to be the teacher of one of their programs called, "Y's Way to a Healthy Back." I excelled at the program because I was using it to treat my own back pain, as well as that of my students who were suffering from back pain as well. I got a lot of positive comments and feedback as a result of teaching that program (see YMCA comment cards in the back of book). Then, the YMCA certified me as a yoga teacher because I developed their yoga program, and trained some of their yoga teachers as well. Now, remember that the YMCA is not in the business of certifying yoga teachers but, because I was a special case, the YMCA of Canada decided to give me a Yoga Certification. So, if you look at my certification, you will see the big YMCA logo on it. I am very proud of that because YMCA is an international organization, which means that my certification should be recognized by all YMCAs worldwide. Allow me to tell you this: the YMCA is the best organization for fitness training. No other organization is better at doing that than the YMCA. Why? Because their mandate is to allow growth of the individual in mind, body, and spirit. They allow you to spread your wings and fly. They will allow you to try anything as long as it's safe, effective, and beneficial. That's what they allow me to do. I was allowed to grow and change yoga to suit a specific demographic of people—and that's people with back pain. I went on to fine tune my yoga, which I called *CorYoga*, to treat back pain—and I became good at it. Then, I went on to create a style of yoga that is specifically for office workers, which I called *Office Yoga Oasis (OYO)*. This is a specific style of yoga that I offer a company's employees to help alleviate back pain, improve productivity, and retard the aging process. So, you see I am using yoga as a tool for treating low back pain.

Does specialized yoga work for treating back pain? In chapter five, you will see what the studies have shown, but let me continue.

You see, when I got my back injury in 1975, it was a bad thing. But that was the thing that led me to exactly where I am today, and I am happy doing what I am doing today—healing people's back pain, especially office workers, through my specialized style of yoga, *Office Yoga Oasis*. I never did become a chiropractor. I flunked out of university; I am not proud of that, but it's the facts. However, I still ended up serving other people by helping to heal their back pain. It's a very satisfying work. My injury was a blessing in disguise.

That which you were not good at, you will become expert at.

That which you consider to be a disadvantage, is your greatest advantage.

Ummm, have you heard or read this somewhere else before? It must be an important statement.

I tell you, the universe has plans for all of us, and if you think you can change those plans, good luck with that!!

If you want to find out what plans the universe has for you (in other words, what you are supposed to do in this lifetime), the best thing you can do is quiet your mind, listen, watch (for signals), and observe—pay attention and all will be revealed to you.

A quick story:

There was this guy, and he was complaining to the Universe. He said,

"Oh, my God, you never answer my prayers; I pray to you constantly but you never answer my prayers." Then, finally, the Universe said,

"I always answer your prayers; no prayers ever go unanswered. I am always giving you what you need even before you ask. I give you what you need, but you are just not paying attention. The next time you pray to me,

Pay attention to the next headline that you read in the newspaper;

Pay attention to the next thing that you hear on the radio;

Pay attention to the next person you pass by on the road;

Pay attention to the next conversation you overhear on the subway in a crowd of people.

Pay attention to the next time you bump your elbow or toes on an object.

Just pay attention because the Universe doesn't always communicate with you in plain, confusing English language.

If you really want to get into close communication with that which you call the Divine, look to see how you feel. This is the best way that the Divine communicates with you.

You see, nothing bad ever happens; these are just ways in which the Universe communicates with you. Sometimes, some of us need to get a big bong over the head in order to pay attention. In my case, I got a big bong in the back. You don't need to bong me twice, I am all bonged out!! I am paying attention now. I accept that I was born to be a back healer.

What about you? Who are you? What work are you here to do?

Your Assignment:

Look back in your life and write out the details of 1 major incident that was a bad thing back then—something that turned out to be a blessing in disguise for you today. Submit it to me at www.backcare world.com.

MY PLAN: When I get enough of these stories, I will put them into a book and publish it in my third book. So, if you want to get your story published, submit them to me at www.backcareworld.com

Do this before you go on to chapter 3.

Lee Downer

I will tell you another story to illustrate how sometimes that which you are absolutely certain is so, given some time, you will come to realize that it is not so; in fact, it is the opposite.

In 1989, I met Kelly at the YMCA. I used to be her trainer. She was pretty, strong, and had many good physical qualities, if you know what I mean. However, there were many things about her personality that I did not like. And I won't tell you what they are because I like my teeth exactly where they are. (But under my breath—driving, domineering, bossy, pushy—

I am just thinking, not saying, just thinking.)

Now if you are thinking that I am suggesting that she would punch my teeth out . . .well, she is not violent, even though she is well trained in martial arts. I am just saying!!

Anyway, as I got to know her, I learned that she had a job that required her to do long distance driving. She would be required to drive several times per week from Toronto to London, Kingston, Ottawa, Montreal, etc. As a result of sitting and doing all that long distance driving, she ended up having a herniated disc (exactly what I had, except I got mine through a traumatic injury while she got hers from sitting too long and driving long distance).

Can you relate to that? Any long distance drivers out there?

So, Kelly and I went through the very same back pain condition—herniated disc and degenerative disc disease, at the lumbar location L4, L5. In fact, she has a tear in that disc, which is another cause of back pain, but you have to wait until you get to chapter 4 to learn how this can cause severe low back pain.

Why does long distance driving cause low back pain?

Because all of the vibration on the road settles in the lower back, causing spinal compression which causes the spinal disc to bulge out, putting pressure on the spinal nerve root, causing pain.

Makes sense? Are we on the same page?

Of course, pun intended! I am not good at humour but I am working on it.

This is how I learned that sitting and driving long distance usually causes back pain, and I have suggestions as to how to alleviate back pain caused by long distance driving.

But wait, let me finish my Kelly story first.

As I learned more about Kelly, I still didn't like her, but we got to be friends. Then, our friendship grew. But I still didn't like her. In fact, I couldn't stand her. I don't know why we became friends. I think it was because we ended up in the same martial arts class together. Then, I start having these internal fights with myself. One day I would like her; the next day I wouldn't like her. I would tell my university buddy, Rick, that I like her; the next day I would tell Rick that I don't like her. I believe if my friend, Rick, goes mental, it's all my fault; I drove my friend crazy with this *I like her, I don't like her* thing. Eventually, Kelly and I fell in love, and I married her in the year 2000. Here is the craziest thing. I asked her to marry me twice, on two different occasions, and she said "NO" both times!

Now, I know what you are thinking again. You are thinking that I am useless when it comes to women. After all, considering no girlfriends or dates in high school, and turned down for marriage twice in adulthood . . . oh, crap, but you know what I mean, right? (Oh, *shit!*) I need help!

I figured three no's is a definite strike out. So I didn't ask her anymore—I just went ahead and married her anyway. Today I can tell you unequally, without the shadow of a doubt, that Kelly is my soul mate, and we both know that. I believe that we must have made an agreement when we were over on the other side, before we came into this life, to meet and be life mates. If you met Kelly today, you would swear that all the words I wrote about her were all lies. But she will tell you that they are all true because today she is nothing of that person I just described above. Today she is kind, caring, sweet, thoughtful, and the most wonderful person I have ever met.

So the person who I couldn't stand, ended up being my soulmate. Who would ever think!! Go figure!! The universe has an amazing sense of humour, so watch for it.

Those who you couldn't stand, you will end up loving.

That which you are not good at, you will become expert at.

Nothing bad ever happens!

Now don't even think of putting this book down. Just race on over to Chapter 3 to start finding out the major causes of back pain.

What are you waiting for?

Go!

Chapter 3

The Causes of Back Pain

Back pain is a complex and personal experience. It can be a very complicated and difficult thing to diagnose. If you have back pain that lasts anywhere up to three months, it is called acute pain. Back pain that lasts more than 3 months is categorized as chronic back pain. This was what I had to live with for 27 years—chronic low back pain.

There are many events that can lead to low back pain. Some of these events are improper bending and twisting, lifting, or turning, and all of these can lead to muscle sprain and ligament strain. Muscle sprain and ligament strain is one of many ways in which you can get back pain. This is what I call *pain caused by tension.*

Tension

What is muscle tension? Tension is tightness—stiff, tight muscles.

A typical scenario:

You are sitting in your office and working on your computer, as so many of us do on a regular basis. You have a deadline to meet and you are working as fast as you can, but time is running out. You have to get the work done or else it may affect company performance, and your boss wouldn't be happy and there may be negative consequences. So, after a few hours you start to notice that your back is getting tight, but you've got to get your work done, so you ignore the tightness and continue to work. The mental tension is building and so is the tightness in your back. By the end of the day, your back is killing you; you are experiencing excruciating back pain. You can't bend because your muscles are restricting your motion. Does any of that sound familiar? I know, because that used to be me. That was my situation when I was a draftsman. Often, I was working under a deadline to get the drawings done in order to make them into manuals to send to the customers so the company could get paid for the equipment that we manufactured for them.

When you have mental or emotional stress, it can manifest itself into your physical body, so your body tenses up. When stress builds in your mind, so too does the stress build in your back muscles, especially in your upper back and neck but not excluding the lower back. For example, when you are startled or frightened, your body tenses up. This is the fight or flight response. It prepares you to fight or run away.

When your back gets tight, your muscles tense and tighten up. When that happens, it restricts your motion, but you need to move, so you move anyway; that can lead to muscle sprain and ligament strain. Tight muscles can also pull on your vertebrae and compress them. Add to that the fact that you have been sitting for a long time in your office; this can cause more compression and tightness. Keeping the back in the same position for long periods of time doesn't help. It is best to rest your back and spine periodically.

So, when the vertebrae are pulled together, caused by tightness, it squeezes the discs, pushing them out and causing them to bulge. When a disc bulges out, it can put pressure on the surrounding spinal nerves, which can cause pain.

What is the best way to deal with this pain caused by muscle tension?

First of all, you must deal with the mental stress. Breathing long, deep, fluidic breaths can calm your mind and lower mental stress.

Secondly, you must stretch out tight muscles. However, the best way I know of dealing with tight muscles is to put them in a warm bath, but since you are at work in your office, and you don't have the luxury of a warm bath, the next best way to deal with these tight muscles is to stretch them out, gently. Stretching out tight muscles is a really good way to alleviate low back pain caused by tightness. That works for me all the time. So, what stretch can you do, and how? One of the easiest and most effective stretches I know for dealing with tight low back muscles is *Standing Forward Bend.* There are others, but this is the easiest and simplest, and it can be done in the comfort of your office without having to change your clothes or needing any special equipment like a yoga mat.

But the ultimate way to deal with a tired back in the office is to lie down flat on your back. As a draftsman, we used to do this all the time during our break time, if we didn't have rush drawings to complete. We used to lie down on the table that we would put the finished drawings on. That was how I became aware of the incredible benefits of lying down on your back in the middle of the workday. You should try it!!

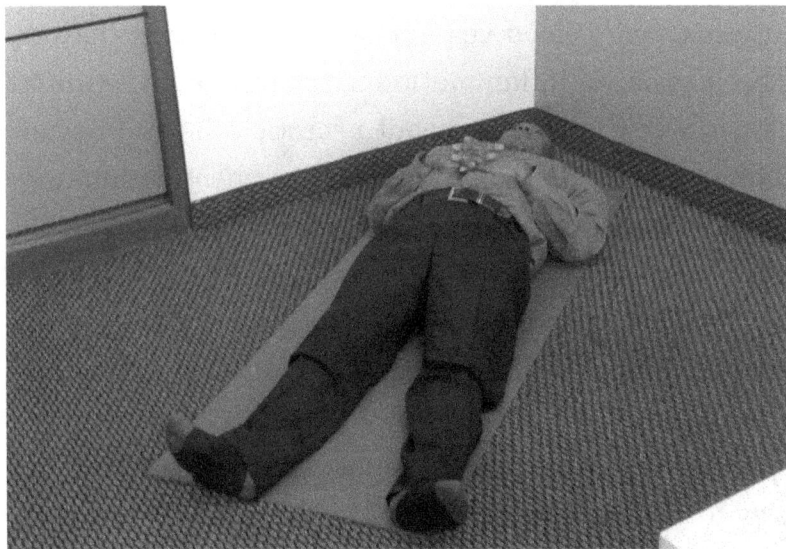

Fig. 1
Photo: Lying down

For your free colour version of this photo, go to
www.backcareworld.com.

Inflammation

What is inflammation?

Inflammation is part of the complex biological response of body tissues to harmful stimuli, such as pathogens, damaged cells, or irritants.

Inflammation is a protective response that involves immune cells, blood vessels, and molecular mediators. The purpose of inflammation is to eliminate the initial cause of cell injury, clear out necrotic cells and tissues damaged from the original insult and the inflammatory process, and to initiate tissue repair.

The classical signs of acute inflammation are pain, heat, redness, swelling, and loss of function.

From my experience, the fastest and most efficient way to treat inflammation is with an anti-inflammatory drug (Your family doctor can prescribe one for you.). The other ways in which I deal with inflammation is by taking a natural anti-inflammatory pill, as well as icing and stretching the body part. Both stretching and icing causes increased blood flow to the area, which flushes the area with blood, which in turn cleans and re-nourishes the area and makes it better.

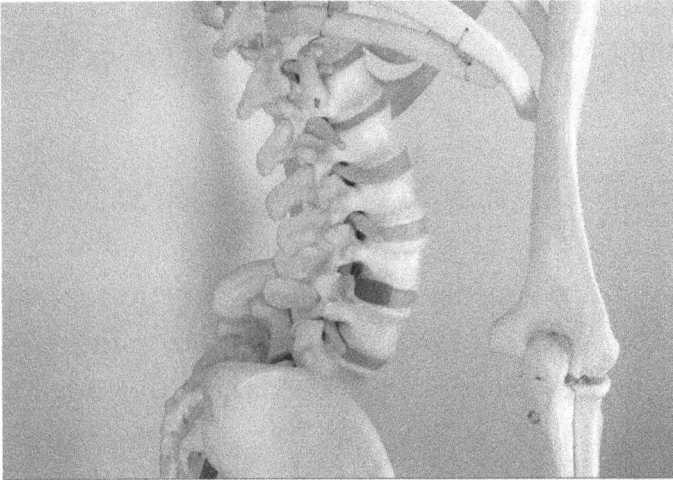

Fig. 2

For your free colour version of this photo, go to

www.backcareworld.com.

Facet Joint Syndrome

Take a look at this figure above. Notice the bones protruding out at the back of the spine. These are called facet joints.

These facet joints in your back are the second most common cause of chronic low back pain. They are joints like your finger, shoulder, and knee joints. They are synovial joints and they have the same basic parts as your hips, knees, and shoulders. However, you can only see them with an X-ray because they are deep in the spine.

Notice how they are close together and they are almost touching each other? These joints tend to be more painful when you stand and extend or bend backwards. Standing puts a lot of load on the facet joints of your spine, and that's why when you stand, they tend to be more painful. So, people who stand for a long time can expect to get facet joint syndrome. Sitting tends to make the pain less. This is a simple test you can perform to determine what may be causing your back pain. If you stand and you feel pain, and when you sit the pain subsides, then you may be experiencing facet joint syndrome. People who experience this kind of back pain are retail workers, sous chefs, or anyone who must stand for prolonged periods of time in their job.

Now that we know what the second most common cause of back pain is, and how it is caused, what can we do about this kind of back pain? Well, take a look at the figure above again and you will notice how close together the bones are. You also know that standing and bending backwards (in this case) puts a lot of load on the joints, and that causes pain, right? Then you would come to the logical conclusion that sitting and bending forward would ease the pain, right? That is the same conclusion that I have come to as well, and guess what? It works! So, if you stand, you need to sit; if you sit, you need to stand. You need to create motion in your spine.

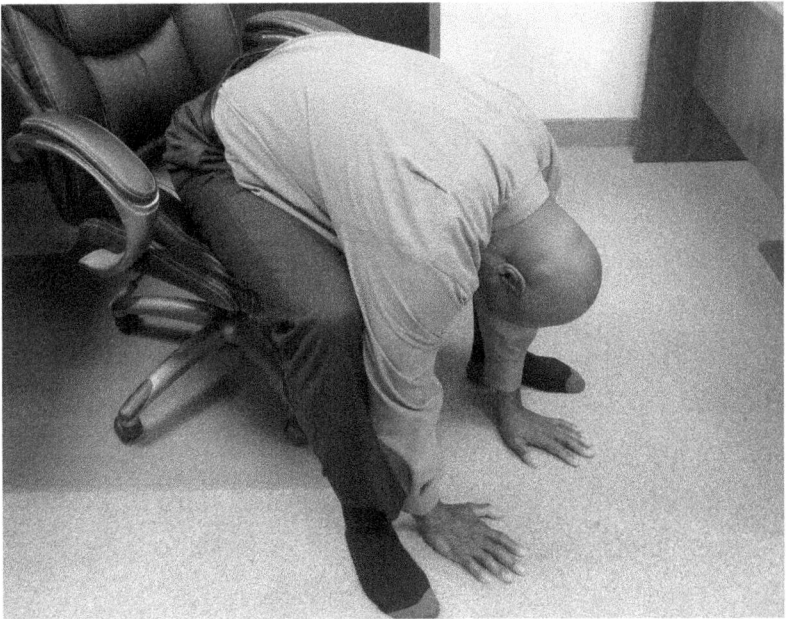

Fig. 3

For your free colour version of this photo, go to
www.backcareworld.com.

If you sit, you need to stand; if you stand, you need to sit.

You may be thinking, "Make up your mind buddy. What kind of mind bending, mumbo jumbo, double talk is this!!"

If you sit for a long period of time, you need to stand and give your back a rest. If you stand for a long period of time, you need to sit and rest your back as well.

Because this book is specific to office workers, and they sit for a long time, I am going to give you nine ways in which prolonged sitting can harm your body.

1. The head

After sitting for too long, blood clots can form and travel to the head. This can result in having a stroke. Get up and get your blood circulation going, and stop playing *head games!*

2. Neck

After a day of long term sitting, fluid that retains in the legs can travel to the neck at night and contribute to sleep apnea. Get up now!

3. Lungs

Prolonged sitting can cause fluid to back up in and *between two lungs* of individuals who experience heart failure. Get moving!

4. Heart

A sedentary lifestyle can contribute to cardiovascular diseases. Get going!! Do it *straight from the heart.*

5. Arm

Physical activity can lead to reduced risk of hypertension and high blood pressure. Let's get the body active. *Let's get it started.* Move it!!

6. Stomach

Sitting for too long can contribute to obesity and colon cancer. Let's get physical and do some crunches for *yo stomach.* Go!

7. Legs

Fluid can collect during prolonged sitting. Walking can pump it out before it causes problems. Get up and get walking from office to office. Do it till your *legs shake!* NOW!

8. Feet

Poor circulation can cause numbness in the feet. Prolonged sitting can cause pressure on your nerves and nerve damage. Get up and get walking because *these feet are made for walking*, and that's just what they'll do. Get going!!!

9. Back

Prolonged sitting places a high amount of pressure on your spine. Over a period of time, the result will be spinal disc compression. Because of the pressure on the tight muscles, any sudden movement can lead to back injury. And your back bone is connected to your hip bone, and your hip bone is connected to your foot bone... get up and get stretching your back until you are *back in the high life again.*

Your Assignment

The titles of some songs are included in the points above. Find the titles of the songs and the names of the artists who made them popular. Go to www.backcareworld.com and submit the titles of the songs and the names of the artists. If you correctly name all the songs and the artists, you will receive a free back care video download.

A quick story

One Saturday morning, I got up and went into the kitchen to make breakfast for my wife (yes, the same Kelly, I only have one) while she slept.

By the time she got up, it was an hour later and I had been standing in the kitchen making breakfast for about an hour. At this point, my lower back was getting really tight—not painful, just really tight. This was restricting my forward bending motion. Can you relate to having tight back as a result of long-term standing? If you can't, go talk to some retail workers and some sous chefs.

Nevertheless, breakfast was cooked and ready for eating.

While waiting for her to wash up, I sat down in a comfortable chair for about 10 minutes to rest my back.

By the time she finished washing up and came to the breakfast table, my back was feeling loose and normal again. Yahoo!!

That was a big lesson for me.

If you stand for a long period of time, you need to periodically sit down, take the pressure off your back, and rest it. This is part of the reason why people (like chefs, security guards, etc.) who spend a long time standing get back aches and pain. They stand and compress their spine, which eventually leads to pain. Imagine if you were a retail worker or a sous chef, standing for 6 or more hours at work; imagine how tight and sore your back would feel during or at the end of the day.

Charles's Story

One of my students is a sous chef, and I remember him telling me that he can remember one time when his back was so painful from standing all day at work that, at the end of his work day, when he got home it took him about 30 minutes just to be able to bend over to untie his shoe laces to take his shoes off.

I feel that it's a crime to have workers stand for a prolonged period of time in their jobs. It's an assault on the human back. You know what is going to happen, right? The workers are going to develop back problems and it will cost them their health, and it will cost the company money.

So, STOP IT!!

Do you want to hear something really interesting? I have never met anyone who had developed back pain and then had it cured. From my experience, once you've developed back pain, it can never be cured. You can manage it to the point where you don't have back pain for many, many years. That's me. But there is always the chance that some form of back pain can come back. So, if you have never had back pain, do whatever it takes to not get it. It breaks my heart when I go into a store and I see their security guards or retail workers standing for so long on their feet and not being able to sit down and rest their back or even bend over to stretch their back. That's a crime! At the end of each day, we are all humans capable of being hurt. I know, because I am coming to you from personal experience! Remember me, "Dead-an-Wake," the kid who almost didn't survive his childhood?

Can we just stop treating these people like they are machines? Treat them well and they will perform well for you and make your company more money! Make sense? Cool? Do it!

In a situation where you work in a position where you stand for a long time, you need to sit down periodically—better yet, lie down.

And conversely, if you sit for a long time in your office, you need to periodically stand up and stretch your back. Better yet, stretch your back and lie down.

So, which is it, sit or stand? The answer is both. Your back and spine needs motion for it to stay healthy.

Doctor Timothy McCall, M.D., *Yoga Journal's* medical editor and board-certified specialist in internal medicine, puts it this way in his article, "Count on Yoga": 38 Ways Yoga Keeps You Fit

- "Spinal disks—the shock absorbers between the vertebrae that can herniate and compress nerves—crave movement. That's the only way they get their nutrients. If you've got a well-balanced asana practice with plenty of backbends, forward bends, and twists, you'll help keep your disks supple."

And this will therefore keep your back and spine healthy.

So, there you have it. Motion is lotion for your spine.

Now, to find out the most common cause of low back pain, fly on over to the next chapter without hesitation.

Chapter 4

Spinal Compression

There are many other ways of getting back pain. However, by far, the most common cause of low back pain is spinal disc problems. Spinal disc problems can cause pain in two ways:

1. Disc herniation
2. Disc tear

Both of these can be attributed to spinal compression.

Spinal compression is the root of most back pain evil.

1. Disc Herniation

The more common of these two is disc herniation, and the major cause of spinal disc herniation is spinal compression.

What is spinal compression?

Spinal compression happens when one object presses down on top of another object. In the case of the spine, you have one vertebra pressing down on top of the vertebra below it. When you sit for a long time, you can compress your spine. If your posture is bad, gravity will accentuate the problem and that can lead to back pain. A good example of people who sit and compress their spine are office workers and drivers. Drivers include bus drivers and, especially, truck drivers. Truck drivers have it the worst because they are stuck sitting in the same position, driving for long hours. What makes matters worse is that all the vibration from the road settles in their lower back, causing even more spinal compression. This is what happened to Kelly (see chapter 2).

Spinal Disc Herniation is when your spinal disc bulges out and puts pressure on the surrounding spinal nerve root; this causes pain. This is what I had for 27 years, but mine was caused by a traumatic injury.

What would cause a spinal disc to bulge out? The most common cause of bulging discs is spinal compression which is caused by prolonged sitting (as in when you sit in your office) or prolonged standing (as in the case of chefs and retail workers). The pain is a result of spinal nerve inflammation, as well as swelling that is caused by the pressure of the disc pressing on the surrounding spinal nerve.

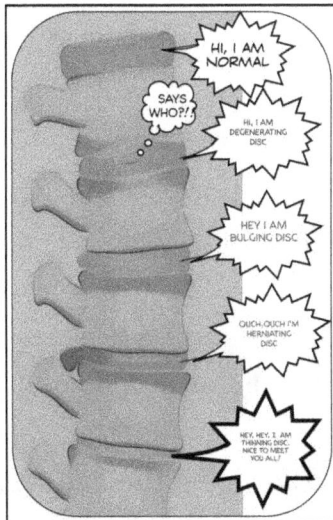

Fig. 1

For your free colour version of this photo, go to

www.backcareworld.com.

Herniated disc is also referred to as bulging disc, or ruptured disc, or slipped disc. I have also heard people describe their back pain as "my back went out." When I hear such things, I often say, "What? How ungrateful and rude. You have lived with your back and taken care of it for all these years, and now it just decides to go out without you, without even asking your permission. How ungrateful and rude."

The lumber spine is where most herniated discs occur. This is where nerves from the spinal cord exit between the lumbar vertebrae and then join together again to form the sciatic nerve. The sciatic nerve runs down your leg.

Lumbar disc herniation is one of the most common causes of lower back pain. They occur 15 times more often than cervical (neck) disc herniation. Cervical (neck) disc herniation occurs 8 % of the time. Upper-to-mid back (thoracic disc) herniation occurs only 1 to 2 % of the time. Why? Because the thoracic spine is supported by ribs that keep the mid spine fairly stable in comparison with the lumbar and cervical spine. When a bulging disc puts pressure on the sciatic nerve, that causes pain down the leg, and that is now called sciatica.

So, as you can see, sciatic pain can be caused from a herniated disc as well.

Sciatica

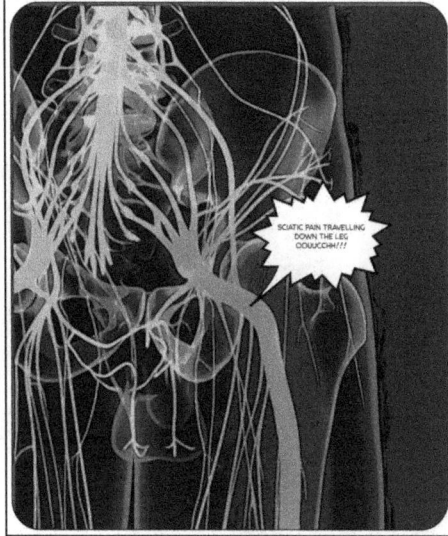

Fig. 2

For your free colour version of this photo, go to
www.backcareworld.com.

Assignment:

Write down the name of one person you know who has sciatica.

So, how do we treat back pain in the office that is caused by spinal compression? Spinal de-compression of course! How do you decompress your spine while in the office? The best way I know of doing that is by doing *Standing Forward Bend*. For details on how to do *Standing Forward Bend* properly, refer to chapter 10.

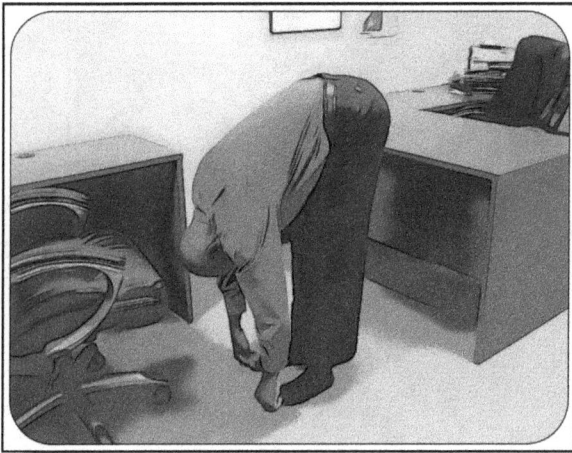

Fig. 3

For your free colour version of this photo, go to

www.backcareworld.com.

2. Disc Tear

As we age, our discs dry out and become hardened. The outer wall of the disc may weaken, and it may no longer be able to contain the gel-like nucleus which contains inflammatory proteins in the centre. When this innermost part of the disc tears, and the gel-like substance (inflammatory proteins) seeps out and irritates surrounding nerves, it causes pain. This is pain caused by disc tear. This is the second most common cause of back pain that is associated with spinal disc.

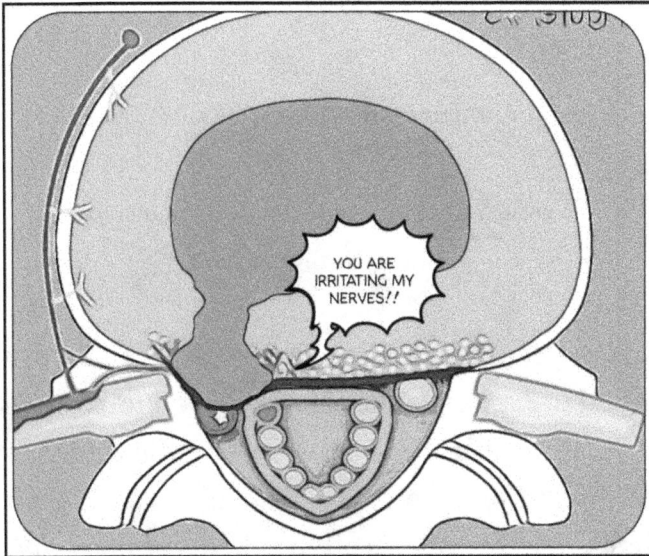

Fig. 4

For your free colour version of this photo, go to
www.backcareworld.com.

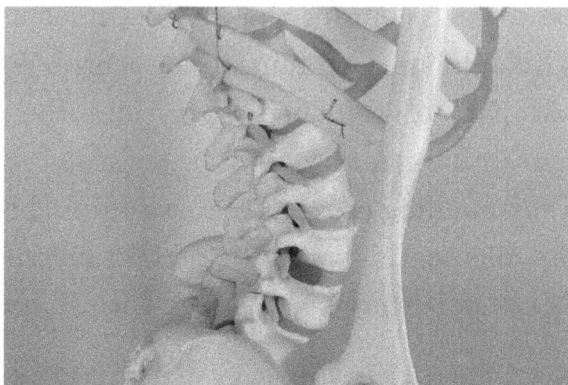

Fig. 5
Compression (Mr. Flexible)

For your free colour version of this photo, go to
www.backcareworld.com.

This is a representation of you when you sit or when you stand for a long time. Notice how the bones of the lower lumbar spine are pressing against each other. Notice the red bulge on the side. This is a bulging disc, herniated disc, or what is often called a *slipped disc*. But discs don't really *slip*; they don't jump out or your spine, walk down the road, step on a banana peel, and slip. That doesn't happen. Discs herniate or bulge.

When you sit for long hours as you do in your office, you compress your spine, the disc bulges out, puts pressure on the spinal nerve, the nerve sends a message to the brain, and the brain sends back a message saying there is pain there in your lower back. This is the most common cause of lower back pain—pain that is caused by spinal disc.

Here is a quote taken from the Journal of the American Academy of Orthopaedic Surgeons, January 2009 issue. (http://www.aaos.org/AAOSNow/2009/Jan/research/research6/)

"Although nonsurgical treatment for back pain is the treatment of choice, when back pain becomes so disabling that patients can no longer function in the activities of daily living, spine surgery may be performed. The three procedures most commonly performed are spinal diskectomy, spinal fusion, and spinal decompression."

Now think this through. If one of the most commonly performed procedures for treating back pain is spinal de-compression, then that would indicate that spinal compression is one of the most common causes of back pain. If the solution is spinal de-compression, then the problem must be spinal compression. Makes sense to me; how about you?

This is spinal de-compression, and he hasn't even gone to full forward bend as in Fig. 6b yet.

The answer from my experience is: *Standing Forward Bend.*

Fig. 6a   *Fig. 6b*

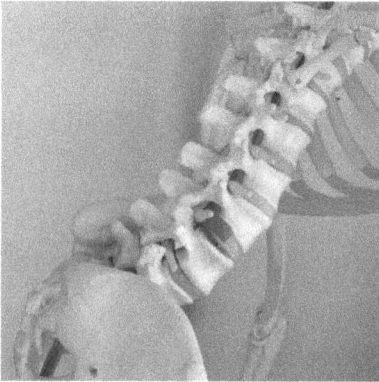 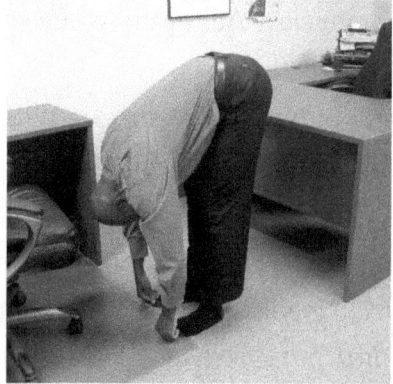

For your free colour version of this photo, go to
www.backcareworld.com.

Take a look at Mr. Flexible in figure 6a. Notice the red object on the side. That is a herniated disc. As well, notice the big gap between the disc, the vertebrae and the nerve. This is spinal de-compression, and he hasn't even gone to full forward bend as in Fig. 6b yet. Now take a look at Fig. 6b and imagine how much greater a spinal de-compression you would be getting if you were to do this. If we all do spinal de-compression on a regular basis, as well as stretch out the muscles around the spine regularly, this will counteract the effects of gravity, allowing us to maintain the length of our spine and alleviate low back pain.

Back Pain

What does back pain feel like?

My experience tells me that there are four main causes of low back pain: inflammation, tension, facet joint syndrome, and compression—and they all feel slightly different. Pain caused by inflammation is sharp; it's nagging, and it lingers. When you move your body in a certain direction, you feel it, but it's not debilitating.

Tension is tightness in the muscles of your back. When you try to move in a certain direction you can't move because your muscles are restricting your motion. And if you force the motion, then you feel sharp pain because then you are tearing your muscles. Facet Joint Syndrome feels similar to muscle tension; it feels tight.

Compression is the most debilitating of the four main causes of back pain from my experience.

Why?

Because compression causes spinal nerve pinch. And what does that feel like?

Here is my experience:

I remember, when I was a teenager, this one time when I was sitting on my mother's couch in the living room and I tried to get up to do something. I can't remember what I was getting up to do because the back pain memories overwhelmed the other memories. In the initiation of the movement to get up, I felt a stab. I call it a stab because that's exactly what it felt like. It felt like someone took an ice pick and thrust it deep into my lower back. And in that moment, I was stopped in my tracks; I was momentarily paralyzed. I couldn't breathe because breathing might have caused another stab. I couldn't move a muscle; all I could do was just hold my breath and hope that the pain would dissipate quickly, which never happened.

It just lingered until I was able to slowly maneuver myself off the couch and onto the floor. There, I would again slowly and gingerly put my lower legs up on the couch in order to ease pressure off my lower back. That was a regular occurrence with me, not just from a sitting position but from a standing position as well.

My back pain continued through to my adulthood. I went on to marry my best friend, Kelly, and, of course, you know we both had the same back pain, caused by a herniated disc and degenerative disc disease.

There was this time when I was experiencing a bad bout of back pain that I was in bed for a whole week. On this one particular day, I was in bed lying down on my back and I needed to go to the bathroom. The simple task of rolling over from my back to my side, which would normally take most people one or two seconds, took me about five minutes. So, finally, I maneuvered myself onto my side. Now, getting from my side to a sitting upright position was another major task; I had to rely on the entire strength of my upper body to push myself up. But another major task faced me again—I couldn't put pressure on my hips to walk. So, my wife bear hugged me and, together, we both stood up with most of my weight on her. Then, we slowly shuffled off to the bathroom. When we got to the bathroom, I held on to the sink (which was close to the toilet) for dear life, with all of my body weight being held by my arms. Then, Kelly slowly released me and pulled down my pants, bear hugged me again, and together we both squatted down—me on the toilet and she in front of me. Once I finished my business, she would bear hug me again and slowly stand up. We would then slowly shuffle off back to the bedroom. When we got there, she would again squat down with me on the bed. She wanted to help me lie down on the bed but she couldn't. It was something that I had to do for myself. I had to slowly and gingerly maneuver myself into a position that didn't cause pain in order to lie down. Then I would slowly gingerly maneuver myself back to a lying down position. That's how I was able to go to the bathroom.

That was one of the many painful situations that Kelly and I went through. So, you see, when someone says to me that they have back pain, I don't just hear what they say—I feel what they say.

But even pain itself is not a bad thing. Pain is the body's protective mechanism. It is a sign of tissue damage. Pain tells you two things:

1. You are alive.

2. You are damaging your body tissue.

So, whenever you have pain, stop whatever it is you are doing that is causing the pain and remedy the situation. But you are going to say to me, "But Lee, you don't understand. I work in an office and my pain is caused from long term sitting. What can I do about that?" You can get up periodically and stretch, and you can lie down. More on that later.

Just remember that pain is a sign of tissue damage. It is not a bad thing; use it as a flag to take care of yourself.

Nothing bad ever happens!

Go to Chapter 5 to find out what they found.

Chapter 5

Research Findings

What They Found

The Cost of Low Back Pain

What are the costs to us for treating low back pain?

According to the website of the *American Academy of Orthopedic Surgeons*, in 2004, the estimated annual direct cost of treating back pain was $193.9 billion. Between 1996 and 2004, the cost of spine conditions increased by 49 percent. The largest share of increase was related to prescription medications. In addition, annual indirect costs for lost wages resulting from back pain were estimated to add another $22.4 billion to this cost, totaling $216.3 billion.

Is that a lot of money? No, it's waaay too much money that we are paying for back pain!!

Equally costly is the impact of back pain on the quality of people's lives. Back pain is the most frequently identified cause of limitation in the ability to work or walk. Between 1999 and 2004, an average of 62 percent of persons reporting work or walking limitations reported low back pain as the cause. Neck pain was the second most frequently cited cause.

In 2004, 25.9 million persons lost an average of 7.2 days of work due to back pain—a total of 186.7 million workdays lost that year.

Is that a lot? You tell me!

216 billion dollars is what it costs to treat back pain. That was in 2004. What is it today? What does it cost your organization as a result of back pain? What does it cost you personally as a result of back pain? The culprit is gravity, and we can reverse it. Gravity, along with prolonged sitting and standing, causes spinal compression. Spinal compression causes disc bulging, which results in back pain. Back pain costs money to treat. But you can decompress your spine to a certain

degree in your office (See the program in chapter 10.). But the ultimate way to decompress your spine is through another program that I have created, called *Danglefit*. That will be my next book; watch for it. But right now you can visit the website at www.danglefit.com

The Research Findings

The Department of Health Sciences at the University of York, in the UK, did a randomized controlled study of *Yoga for Healthy Lower Backs* in 2011. It was the largest trial to date into the effectiveness of yoga as a treatment for chronic and recurring low back pain. Basically, 313 adults, aged 18-65 years old, were recruited from 39 GP practices in Cornwall, London, Manchester, and York. They were allocated to either the yoga group (n=156) or usual care group (no yoga) (n=157).

Basically, those in the yoga group did a specialized yoga that is specific for healthy backs, while the usual group did no yoga. During the 12 months studied, those in the yoga group had an average of only 3.83 days off work compared to 12.29 in the non-yoga group (usual care).

Did you get that, office managers and executives?

This is an average saving of 12.29 days - 3.83 days = 8.46 days. In percentage that turns out to be 8.46 days saved/12.29 days lost = 0.688 X 100% = 68.84% days saved or worked by the yoga group. So the yoga group saved 69% of the days lost by the non-yoga group. That means that the people who did yoga were able to work 69% more days compared to the non-yoga group. If they were able to work 69% more of the time than the non-yoga group, that means that they were being potentially 69% more productive than the non-yoga group. Make sense?

Based on this study, we could say that people who do a specialized yoga for back pain are potentially 69% more productive than people who don't do specialized yoga for back pain.

You still with me?

Now let's take that information from this UK study and apply it to our North American study. From the *Journal of the American Academy of Orthopedic Surgeons*, based on a 2004 study, North America lost a total of 186.7 million workdays that year. What if we were to let these people do specialized yoga for healthy backs and were able to save 69% of those 186.7 million days lost?

Shall we do the math?

Let's do it!

186,700,000 days lost X 69% days saved or worked = 128,823,000 days saved. How much more productive would North Americans be if we all worked an additional 128.8 million more days per year?

Alright, maybe that's not so easy to see, so let's look at it from another angle. If we add up the annual direct cost of treating back pain, which is $193.9 billion, with the annual indirect cost of treating back pain, which is $22.4 billion, we have a total of $216.3 billion. What if we were to save 69% of that each year? That would be a saving of $216.3 billion X 69% = $149.3 billion each year. And exactly what would we have to do in order to save all that money? Simply do a specialized yoga that is specific to treating chronic and recurring low back pain. That would be in accordance with the conclusion drawn by the University of York study.

Their conclusion goes as follows: 'On the basis of this trial, 12 weekly group classes of specialized yoga is likely to be a cost-effective intervention for treating patients with chronic or recurrent low back pain.'

After further analyzing the health economic data from the study, they also found and summarized that yoga would most likely be cost-effective both within the UK National Health Service and within society.

So what would a specialized yoga like that look like?

For starters, that would have to be a yoga that is specific to treating back pain conditions. It would be specific to stretching and decompressing the back and spine. It would most definitely have to be something that older adults can do, and not just yoga that only young, flexible, bendy teenagers can do. If it was a yoga that could be done in the comfort of your office, that would be good. If it was short enough to be manageable timewise, yet still be effective, that would be even better. With a program like that, employees could do it regularly and consistently, and thereby being able to alleviate, if not eliminate, their back pain all together.

I have news for you. SUCH A PROGRAM EXISTS!!

It's called *No Pain, Your Gain – How to alleviate back pain and increase productivity*, and you have the book in your hands. The video program is available online at www.backcareworld.com

OK, let's look at a few more studies just to make sure we have enough variety to back up what I am saying.

2. Another study entitled: *Evaluation of the Effectiveness of Iyengar Yoga Therapy on Chronic Low Back Pain*

Ninety subjects were randomized to either the yoga group or the control group. Basically, the yoga group received yoga while the control group received only standard medical care (no yoga).

Results: 'Significantly greater reduction in functional disability and pain intensity were observed in the yoga group when compared to the control group at 24 weeks. Depression was also significantly lower in yoga subjects.'

Conclusion: 'Yoga improves functional disability, pain intensity, and depression in adults with chronic low back pain. There was also a clinically important trend for the yoga group to reduce their pain medication (which costs Americans many billions of dollars per year) usage compared to the control group.'

For yoga and depression, see Erin's story in chapter 8, CorYoga is a Tool.

Next study:

3. Effect of Iyengar Yoga Therapy for Chronic Low Back Pain, 2005

In this US study, a total of 60 participants were randomized equally between a yoga group and educational group. The yoga group received 16 weeks of weekly 90 minute classes of specialized Iyengar Yoga. The educational group received 16 weekly back care newsletters.

Yoga participants were asked to practice at home for 30 minutes, 5 times a week.

At the end, the resulting analyses showed significant reductions in pain intensity (64% reduction), functional disability (77% reduction), and pain medication usage (88% reduction) in the yoga group at the post-intervention 16 week.

I could provide more studies, but it's more of the same.

Basically, it works!!!! Yoga is a solution for low back pain.

A specialized yoga for treating back pain is cost effective in treating chronic and recurring low back pain.

So, what is specialized yoga and where can one find such a program?

Well, if I didn't have a program for you, it would be like telling you that there is an effective treatment for your lower back pain and I have it, but I am not going to tell you or give it to you. Naaa na na nah naahhh!! That would be cruel. And I don't feel like being cruel—not today.

For the simple program, go to chapter 10. For the video program, go to www.backcareworld.com.

Flip over to chapter 6 for how to treat back pain conditions.

Chapter 6

Treating Back Pain Conditions

There is a wide range of treatment that may or may not work for the same kind of back pain condition. It is a personal experience. Remember that this book is written from my own 27 years of experience with back pain, as well as what I have observed and learned from my friends, family, and students. But having said that, if you don't have a broken bone in your back, or if you don't have fused vertebrae, then yoga is most likely the solution for your back pain, as you can see from the research findings in chapter 5.

Based on a CBC news clip, "The science on lower back pain," there is only one method of treatment that has ever been proven effective in reducing the reoccurrence of lower back pain. Of all the other methods of treatments, products, and services that have been advertised and promoted, and have claimed to alleviate low back pain, the only one that has been proven to help alleviate back pain, by as much as 40 %, is still a physical exercise program combined with education. But not all exercise works for alleviating back pain. For example, deadlifts and squats will not help; they will only aggravate low back pain, making it worse. The type of exercise that works is through a stretching exercise program. This has been proven in university studies (see chapter 5, Research Findings). But again, not just any type of stretching exercise will work for alleviating back pain. It has to be a type of yoga. And again, not all types of yoga work for alleviating back pain. For example, Ashtanga yoga (a rigorous and challenging type of yoga) would more likely aggravate a back problem rather than alleviate it. It has to be a type of yoga that is specific to treating and caring for the back. And for people who are working in the office, it would ideally be something that they could do while at their desk—a type of yoga that is manageable timewise yet effective.

Once again, based on the *Journal of the American Academy of Orthopaedic Surgeons* website, the three procedures most commonly performed for treating back pain are spinal diskectomy, spinal fusion, and spinal decompression.

If spinal decompression is a treatment, then what's the cheapest, most effective way to decompress the spine, especially when you are in your office?

One answer is: Standing Forward Bend.

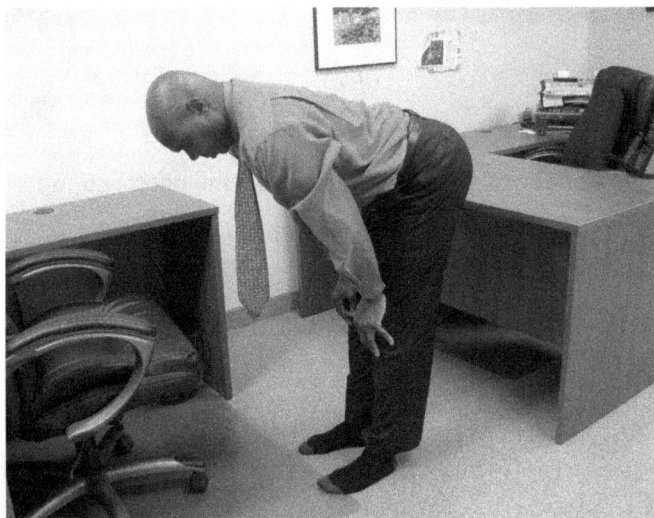

Fig. 1

For your free colour version of this photo, go to
www.backcareworld.com.

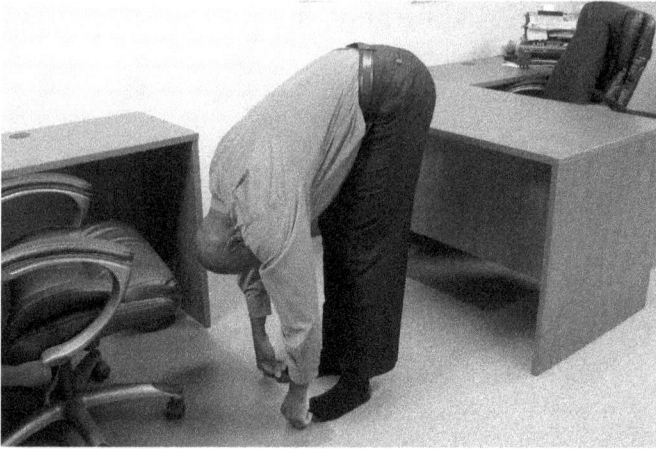

Fig. 2

For your free colour version of this photo, go to
www.backcareworld.com.

1. Anti-inflammatory Drugs

How do you know if it is inflammation or spinal compression that is causing your back pain? You don't know because they feel the same. Compression usually causes bulging of the disc, which irritates the nerve. Inflammation also disturbs the nerve root. But compression can lead to inflammation. So, if you are experiencing that sharp stabbing pain, then I would suggest taking an anti-inflammatory drug, just to be safe, to alleviate the tenderness; then, as soon as the tenderness subsides, jump head first into yoga to decompress the spine and loosen up the tight muscles around the area on a regular basis.

The best way I know of dealing with inflammation is by taking an anti-inflammatory drug. Now, please don't get me wrong; I am not advocating or promoting the use of drugs. However, I have discovered that sometimes the things that you don't want to do are exactly the things that you need to do. For example, who wants to take some drugs? Not me! But sometimes you need to take some anti-inflammatory drugs in order to deal with the inflammation that is happening right now. So, get some from your family doctor. But as soon as the pain subsides or has gone away, you need to dive into yoga. You must do whatever it takes to keep your back loose, strong, flexible, supple, and healthy, because If your back doesn't work, then you don't work.

2. Ice

When people with back pain ask me what I do for torn muscles, I tell them I sleep on ice. They tend to look at me like I am crazy and start laughing. Then, I think, "Better you laugh at me than me be you, cause I don't have back pain, but you do."

Whenever I go to work out at the gym, I often like to sleep on ice that night. Why? Because weight training causes minute tears in your muscles, including the back muscles. Those minute muscle tears can cause the back to ache and pain. One very effective way to treat that is to put ice on the back, so I sleep on a frozen ice gel pack. Some people ask, "Doesn't that cause frost bite?" No, because when you lay down on the frozen gel pack, after some time, the frozen gel pack will become warm because you have more heat in your body than there is cold in the gel pack. So, eventually, the frozen gel pack will become warmer and warmer as the night goes on, so it presents no danger to your body at all. Here is the benefit of putting ice on your body: you are a warm blooded person and your body wants to be warm. When you put ice on a body part, it restricts blood flow to that area. Your body doesn't like that. The longer your body stays on the ice, the more the ice will melt or get warmer and, therefore, you are effectively removing the ice. When that happens, your body flushes that area with a greater volume of blood. This added blood volume will flush the area with fresh oxygen and nutrients. This will re-nourish the area and make it better. Does that make sense to you? This is how ice therapy works.

3. Massage

I personally find massage therapy to be more effective than chiropractic treatment for treating back issues that is soft tissue related. I remember one time having a really tight back and, after going to get only one treatment of massage, the next day my back was so loose that I was back to normal. The reason why I find massage more effective than chiropractic treatment is because time is spent working on my back, loosening up the tight muscles, leaving them loose and pliable and full of blood. And remember that blood is magic in the body because it brings fresh oxygen and nutrients to re-nourish the area and make it better.

4. Stretching (OYO Videos)

The best way to alleviate and avoid low back pain is to stretch. Why is it that the moment that someone hurts their back and are experiencing low back pain, the first thing that they tend to do is bend over to stretch, even people who don't believe in yoga or stretching?

Do they know instinctively that this is good for them and this is what they need to do? Absolutely!! We all know this instinctively. It's like bumping your elbow.

The moment you bump your elbow, the first thing that you do is put your hand on it and cup the elbow as if you know that hands have healing power. And you do know innately that there is healing power in your hands, just as you know innately that bending is healing for low back pain.

But not all bending is the same. When you bend forward, you need to first lengthen the spine or you may further compress the spine during the bending motion. Did you know that back pain rarely ever occurs while bending sideways or backwards? Take a look at Mr. Flexible again and notice that just the way the vertebrae are, you run a higher risk of compressing the spine and causing back pain if you don't first lengthen and elongate the spine. That's why every time I have people do a forward bend, I first make them reach their arms up as far as they can to make sure that the spine is lengthened before folding forward into a forward bend.

If you are currently experiencing low back pain, and your back is tender, don't even think about doing any stretching or exercise program. When you are in pain the way that I have been, your back is tender and sensitive, and you are not able to do any exercising. At times, I wasn't even able to stand to walk to the bathroom, much less do bending. So, wait until the sensitivity and tenderness has subsided or is gone. You may even find that an anti-inflammatory drug may help with inflammation if that is what is causing your current back pain. When the sensitivity and tenderness is gone, that's the time to jump into the program and do it regularly and consistently, and you may find that your back pain may disappear, never to return. That's what I have experienced. If you wait until your back is in pain to do something about it, you will find that your back pain will always reoccur and will never go away for good. Remember that an ounce of prevention is worth a pound of cure. But if you take action while your back is not in pain, you will find that a long time will go by without you noticing any back pain. That will be because you have properly managed and cured— I mean cared for— your back and spine.

Having said that allows me to tell you this: once you have developed back pain, my experience is that you cannot cure low back pain, BUT you can manage it to the point where you never get back pain for many years. That is me. I haven't had any back pain since 2002, up to this day in 2016, and that is because I have learned to manage it so well that back pain is not a problem for me now. That is why I am able to write this book to teach you how to manage and alleviate your back pain as well.

Some of the best stretches that you can do to heal your lower back pain is back bend, side bend, forward bend, and twisting. This is the basis of my back pain solution.

Doctor Timothy McCall, M.D., *Yoga Journal's* medical editor and a board-certified specialist in internal medicine, puts it this way in his article, "Count on Yoga": 38 Ways Yoga Keeps You Fit

- "Spinal disks—the shock absorbers between the vertebrae that can herniate and compress nerves—crave movement. That's the only way they get their nutrients. If you've got a well-balanced asana practice with plenty of backbends, forward bends, and twists, you'll help keep your disks supple."

Updoggie Downdoggie

I have come to the realization, as you too must have also come to realize, that things are not always what they appear to be.

For example, the two key yoga postures that I believe were extremely instrumental in healing my chronic back pain for good was the *upward facing dog* and *downward facing dog* postures. The upward facing dog is actually a back bend, while the downward facing dog is a forward bend.

Look at the downward facing dog below.

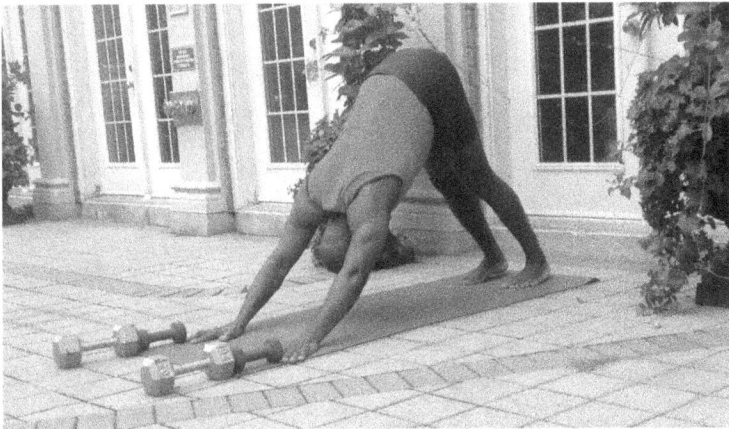

Fig. 3

For your free colour version of this photo, go to
www.backcareworld.com.

In this position, you are pressing your heals toward the ground, you are pressing your tail bone up towards the sky, and you are pressing your shoulders down towards the ground. So, in this posture, you are stretching out the entire back side of your body. You are stretching from your Achilles, calves, hamstrings, and lower, middle, and upper back, and your shoulders. But the most important thing that you are doing for your back in this posture is you are decompressing your spine. You are pushing the vertebrae apart and creating space between your vertebrae for the herniated disc to go back into place where it belongs.

Look at the pictures below of the upward facing dog position.

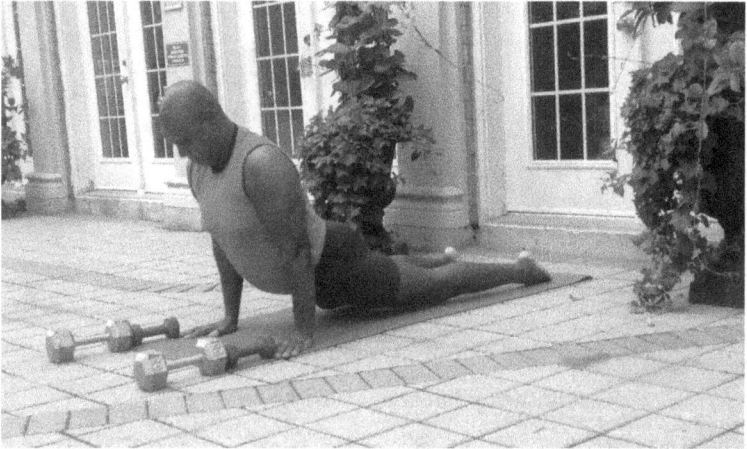

Fig. 4

For your free colour version of this photo, go to
www.backcareworld.com.

In this position your hands are just outside of your chest and under your shoulders. Your arms are straight and your shoulders are pressing backwards and downwards. You are pressing your chest and sternum up towards the sky, and your hips are slightly off the ground.

Look at what is happening in the bones of your lower back during this upward facing dog posture, and notice how the vertebrae looks like they are going to crush each other. In fact, newcomers to yoga who do upward facing dogs usually complain that it feels like they are crunching their back. And a small percentage of these people say that they experience some pain during the upward facing dog. So, here is what I believe happens. When you have a herniated disc and you do upward facing dog, you are actually putting pressure on the disc (thus the pain), but you are also forcing it back into place where it belongs. After doing this posture for some time, you actually work the herniated disc back into place, alleviating the pressure from your nerve root and alleviating your back pain long term. After a while of doing this posture, it actually becomes so comfortable that you will feel like you want to spend more time in this posture, just rocking back and forth.

So, a combination of these postures—the up dog and the down dog—are perfect for forcing herniated discs back into place and alleviating low back pain. These are the two key postures that I believe to be instrumental in healing not only *my* herniated disc but that of the rest of my students as well. So, something that seems like it should cause pain, actually helps to get rid of pain. And, like I said, looks are often quite deceiving.

The Low Back Pain Prevention Program

Let's take a look at some bending and twisting postures and how they help keep the back healthy and pain free.

Spinal Twist

One of the best ways that I know of to keep the spine in proper alignment is to do a type of yoga posture called *spinal twist*.

I remember this one time when a new student came to class and, before I started the class, she came up to me and told me that she had a back problem and that there are certain postures she cannot do. I asked what the nature of her back problem was. She said she had a herniated disc, and her physiotherapist told her not to do any backward bending or twisting of the spine. I thought, "Uummm!! That is exactly what you need to do, but I guess your physiotherapist knows your situation better than I do." Then I said to her, "Well, you can stay and see what we do and how we do it, and if you don't feel it's for you, then you can stay and watch, or you can leave." About three minutes after I started the class, she left.

I remember having another conversation with a student in the change room one evening after another class in a different location.

He said to me, "Lee, do you know what's funny and interesting?"

I said, "What, Charles?"

He said, "The things that you make us do in class that help my back are the exact same things that the physiotherapists will tell you not to do." I said, "What do you mean?"

He said, "My physiotherapist told me never to do any twisting of my back, in any way shape or form, because the spine was not meant for twisting. But that's exactly what helps my back—those twisting exercises that you make us do.

Then he said, "Do you know how I know this? I said, "No, how do you know this?" He said, "Because my physiotherapist is my sister, and she couldn't help me with my back pain, but you did with your CorYoga twisting postures." I said, "Thank you for sharing that; I appreciate you sharing that with me."

So, what should it be? To twist, or not to twist; that is the question.

One of the best ways I know of to keep the spine in proper alignment is to do a type of yoga posture called a spinal twist.

It is what the baseball players do.

It is what the hockey players do.

It is how a chiropractor adjusts you.

It is what the golfers do. Heck, it is the only thing that the golfers do in performing his or her sport! It is an extremely important movement for many sports. Imagine if you were to play a sport and you couldn't twist your spine at all. What would that be like?

Here is what I know about the body. If you spend a long time not doing something that is natural for your body, you will get weak at doing that thing. Then, one day, when you accidentally do that movement, you will be too weak at that angle and, therefore, you will hurt your body. For example, if you never practice twisting your body, your body will get weak at the twisting angle. Then, one day, when you go out and golf, you will injure your back and spine. So, what they say you should not do is exactly what you should do, but carefully and under full control.

The concept of the spinal twist is to realign the spine on a regular basis so that the body can function optimally and, therefore, do what it needs to do to heal itself and maintain proper health.

In fact, the spinal twist is exactly what the chiropractor does to you when you get an adjustment. They make you lie on your side and, carefully and in full control, they very quickly twist your spine. This adjusts and realigns your spine, but a CorYoga twist is much more beneficial than a chiropractor twist because a CorYoga spinal twist not only adjusts the spine and brings it back into alignment, it also stretches and strengthens the muscles along the spine, keeping the spine loose, supple, and strong, on a regular basis. When these muscles are loose and supple, they stop pulling on the spine; this reduces tension and pain, if not eliminating pain all together. Does that make sense to you? It had better, because it makes sense to me.

What is a spinal twist?

A spinal twist is when the upper body (including the shoulders) rotates in one direction while the lower body (including the hips) rotates in the opposite direction. See fig. 5 below (spinal twist)

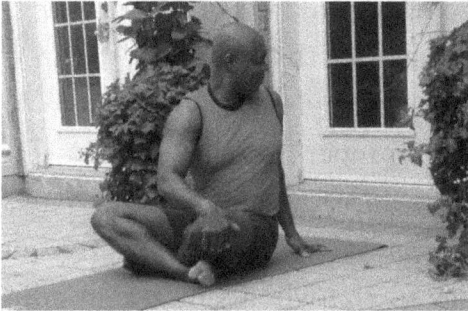

Fig. 5

For your free colour version of this photo, go to

www.backcareworld.com.

There are many types of spinal twists. There are standing twists, bending twists, kneeling twists, sitting twists, and lying twists.

There is also a neutral twist, tuck and twist, and extended twist. All these versions of the twist affect various parts of the spine. For example, while a chiropractor usually adjusts a specific part of the spine, a CorYoga twist will affect the entire spine, because we do many variations of the spinal twist.

So, what are the benefits of a spinal twist?

Well, for starters, it adjusts your vertebrae and realigns your spine, which alleviates pressure from your nerve. This facilitates proper nerve function to your internal organs, which in turn allows them to function optimally. Another major benefit of the spinal twist is that it also stretches the muscles that contribute significantly to lower back pain. Some of these muscles are the multifidus, the longissimus, and the quadratus lumborum.

The spinal twist also squeezes and massages your internal organs, thereby causing increased blood flow to your organs. This increased blood flow brings fresh nutrients, which nourish the organs and improve overall health. Some spinal twists, particularly the prayer twist, will squeeze the entire abdominal region, thereby forcing food stuff through. So this is absolutely great for digestion and elimination. Another major benefit of the spinal twist is that it calms and soothes the central nervous system. The next time you do a spinal twist, pay attention to how your entire body goes calm and quiet.

All hockey players, golfers, and baseball players should do spinal twists regularly and consistently. Why? Because it's a sport specific movement. Their sport requires them to twist their spine. Consider this: if you are a golfer, the most important sport specific move you can do to help improve your game is a spinal twist—you should do it regularly and consistently. Why? Think about this: what sport specific activity does the great Usain Bolt, the fastest man in the world, do?

He runs. Right?

Right! You are thinking, "Yeah, Lee, Daaaaa!!"

That's exactly what I am thinking. "Daaaaa!"

Hockey players, golfers, and baseball players should all do spinal twists.

You wouldn't make Usain play golf in preparation for a race, would you? No! You would make him run, because it's sport specific. Similarly, you should make golfers, hockey players, and baseball players twist their spines regularly and consistently in preparation for their games. Why? Because twisting is sport specific for these players. So, when any professional says not to twist your spine, l cannot agree with that.

Why do sport specific activities? Because it prepares your body for the activity of your sport, so that when you do your actual sport, your body is well used to the movement, so you don't injure yourself but perform with great ease and proficiency.

Chapter 7

Siesta at Work

A hundred and fifty years ago, slave masters would buy slaves and work them to death—literally. Then they would go out, buy more slaves, and again work them to death—and the cycle goes on and on.

Today, large corporations hire employees and work them to ... well, until they quit. Then they would go out, hire more employees, and again work them until they quit—and the cycle continues.

Is there a pattern here? I am just saying! Hashtag!!

How much does it cost your company to go find an employee, train them, and bring them up to company standard? What does it cost your company in lost time and productivity while they are searching for a new employee? I don't know what it costs your organization, but from the "Small Business Employee Benefits and HR Blog," Zanebenefits.com website, here is what they have to say on this matter. The cost of employee turnover seems to vary by wage and role of employee. For example, a study of the Centre for American Progress (CAP) found that the average costs of replacing an employee are:

3. 16% of the annual salary for low paying jobs with a high-turnover rate. These jobs are usually under $30,000 per year. For example, it would cost $3,328 to replace a $10 per hour retail employee.

4. 20% of the annual salary for a middle range position. These would be people who earn between $30,000 and $50,000 per year. For example, it would cost $8,000 to replace a manager who is earning $40,000 per year.

5. Up to 213% of the annual salary for a highly educated individual in an executive position. For example, it would cost $213,000 to replace a CEO making $100,000 per year.

So, you can see that it would cost a company much more to replace an executive than it would be to just keep them and treat them well.

What does this "I don't care about my employees" kind of behavior produce? Well, one thing that it produces for sure is disloyalty. Employees will not be loyal to employers who don't care about their health, and eventually they will leave, if not by force, then by their own choice. Deep down, we all know that our health is our wealth. I know this because at one time I was an employee working in an office.

So, what did I do while I was working in the office? When I was a draftsman, we had a big long table that we would keep finished drawings on. My colleague and I would take turns lying down on the table to rest our backs. It did wonders for me.

If an employee is sitting or standing all day and compressing his spine which causes low back pain, and the employer will not allow the employee to do something to alleviate the pain, eventually that employee will need therapy in order to alleviate the back pain. Make sense? If the employer does not pay for the employee's therapy, then the employee must pay for the therapy, which drains money away from the employee. If the employer chooses to pay for the therapy, then that drains money away from the employer. You still with me? Either way, the back pain costs money—and this can all be avoided.

If the employer does not show caring for the employee's health, then eventually the employee will quit. I did! That cost the employer even more in terms of going out to find, interview, and hire a new employee, as well as train them and bring them up to company standard; plus, add to that, lost productivity, etc. Why not just treat the employee well in the first place and save all that lost time and money?

What does "treat employee well" mean? It means doing whatever it takes to avoid and alleviate back pain. It means providing them with the opportunity for them to alleviate back and neck pain caused from long term sitting and standing. That could mean providing them with the opportunity to take part in a video program at work that will lead them through a back care stretching program. It also means providing them with the opportunity to lay down flat on their back in the middle of the day to rest their tired back.

The absolute best things that you can do while at work to alleviate a tired and painful back is to stretch your back and lie down, and maybe have a mini siesta.

Lying down in the middle of a busy and stressful day is the most incredibly relieving thing you can do. There is nothing like lying down on your back, in the middle of the day, at work, when you are experiencing stress. It is the most incredible stress relieving, rejuvenating act of kindness you can do for your body. Nothing compares to it. Lying down on your back for 2 to 5 minutes will completely de-stress your entire body, rest tired muscles, especially of the back and spine, increase blood blow to your head so you can think clearer, and completely refresh and rejuvenate your entire body. If you are a company executive, wouldn't you want your people to be calm, clear thinking, level headed, and reasonable, especially when going into a negotiation? Then why not provide them with the opportunity to do so? Give them the tools to do what they do best, so that they can perform at their best, so as to improve company's productivity and profitability.

Make sense?

Cool!!

Imagine this: you have been sitting and working for several hours. Your back is tight and painful, and you are stressed.

On your break, you stop to do some simple yet effective yoga stretches. I recommend you do the ones in this book (chapter 10) because these are designed specifically for this purpose, or you can find the video series program at my website www.backcareworld.com. Then you spread out your yoga mat or towel on the floor. Then you sit down, and then lie down on your back. But, before your back hits the floor, you breathe in, and the moment your entire back hits the floor, you breathe out and try to completely empty your lungs with your eyes closed.

The moment your back hits the mat, your body dissolves and completely surrenders into the floor. You inhale deeply, and exhale a big, long sigh of relief. How does your body feel as you exhale?

Loose, stress-free, pain-free, light, a sense of floating?

This is what you can have by lying down in the middle of your workday!

Some employers might argue that having employees lie down while at work would lower productivity, as they may fall asleep. Studies have shown the opposite to be true.

Well, consider this and tell me which part of this makes sense to you: a company that wants to improve productivity and profitability would allow employees to go for a 10 minute "cigarette" break (I have nothing against smokers) but won't let employees take a 10 minute "lie down" break. Does that make sense? One of these activities is productive and one is not. As a company leader, which one would you choose? Which one should you choose? I am not saying that employees shouldn't get "cigarette" breaks; I am just saying that employers should encourage employees to take "lie down" breaks as well.

So, what if large corporations would just encourage their employees to take breaks and lie down and have a 15 minute siesta? What would that do?

This is what would happen: employees would get a sense that employers do care about them, regardless if they do or not. It would create loyalty because these employees would want to stay with companies that show that they care about their employees.

Following the Jumpers

If you look at the action of a long jumper or a high jumper, you will notice that before they start the running process, they will usually take one step backwards in order to propel themselves forward. That technique obviously works as you can see how successful most jumpers are. Successful elite athletes know this and use it, but it seems many corporate organizations don't know this. The concept is: sometimes you need to take a step backwards in order to propel yourself further forward. If you sit or stand at work, you need to stop work and rest your back.

The story goes like this: two tree cutters engaged in a competition to see who could cut down the most trees in one hour. At the start of the competition, they both ran out and started chopping like mad, crazy guys. After about fifteen minutes, competitor A stopped and ran into the forest for ten minutes. Then he came back out and continued cutting down trees. He continued with this behavior every fifteen minutes for the entire hour. At the end of the competition, it was discovered that he won the competition by cutting down the most trees. At the end, in an interview, he was asked what he was doing when he would run off into the forest every fifteen minutes. He answered, "I was sharpening my ax." You see, if you are the executive of a company with employees, and you want them to improve productivity, you need to get them to sharpen their ax every so often. They need to take a step backward in order to propel themselves forward—like a high jumper. They need to sharpen their ax in order to cut down more trees—like the tree cutter. They need to take a back break in order to be more productive. What is a "lie down" break? Make them lie down for five minutes.

If a company will allow their employees to take 5 to 10 minutes to go for a coffee break or a smoke break, doesn't it make sense to encourage them to do something that will help to improve their health, improve productivity, and eventually profitability? Doesn't that make sense? So, why are they not doing it? Because they don't know that this will help. Because to know and not to do, is not to know. So, now I am telling you. Encourage your employees to take a 5 minute break and rest their back by lying down under their desk at work, twice a day.

Here are some additional benefits of lying down during the day at work and having a mini siesta:

- It decompresses the entire spine.
- It gives the muscles of your back a chance to rest and rejuvenate.
- It improves productivity by over 30%.
- It improves alertness by up to 100%.
- It reduces stress and the risk of heart disease by 34%.
- It increases blood flow to your head, which causes you to think clearer and in turn increases negotiation and communication skills.
- It reduces the risk of accidents at work and on the road.
- It increases happiness and wellbeing.
- It reduces physical stress.
- It increases energy.
- It creates employee loyalty.

So, why wouldn't a company encourage their employees to lie down at work for 15 minutes during the work day? Heck, it doesn't even have to be on company time; it could be on the employee's break or lunch time.

Now you are thinking, "Lee, you are asking me to lie down at work? My boss would fire me." But that is a North American mentality. In North America, we tend to think "work, work, work." No rest, just work.

But in other parts of the world, people actually take 2 to 3 hours in the middle of the day to go home and have a nap. In some parts of the Caribbean and Mexico, they do that. In Spain and Italy, they call it *siesta*. Are they any less productive than we are in North America? Don't answer that, considering the current state of the European economy. But all jokes aside, I don't think so. It has been proven that taking a nap in the middle of the day is more productive than not. And there is a list of famous people who regularly take a nap throughout the day.

Here is a list of famous people who took a siesta regularly, and the benefits of napping:

- Bill Clinton napped while President of the United States. It helped him cope with the pressures of the presidential office.
- Brahms napped at the piano while composing his famous lullaby.

- Napoleon napped between battles while sitting on his horse.
- Churchill maintained that he had to nap in order to cope with his wartime responsibilities.
- Geniuses such as Edison and da Vinci all took naps.
- Margaret Thatcher took naps in order to be at her best.
- Einstein would sit in his favorite armchair with a pencil in his hand and doze off. He would then wake when the pencil dropped, ensuring that he did not enter a deep sleep from which it would be difficult to wake up. Napping frequently during the day helped Einstein think more clearly.

So, there are some of the famous people who napped, and some of the benefits. So, why can't we in North America nap throughout the day? Ok, so let's not nap; how about just letting our employees lie down for a few minutes throughout the day and rest their backs while at work. That can only help, not hurt. I highly encourage it!

And here is one final point about lying down and napping throughout the day. If you don't buy into the benefits and the people listed above, then at least consider this: how much does back pain cost your organization each year in terms of time taken off work, hospital stays, and insurance (WSIB) claims? So compare that with the 15 minutes taken off just to lie down and rest their back. And finally, if you still don't buy into any of this, then consider this: your employees are already taking 15 minutes for a coffee break; all you have to do is encourage them to use the time wisely by insisting that they lie down during the day. Try it. You have nothing to lose except stress and back pain, and have much to gain—improved productivity and happy, healthy, loyal employees. At least you will have happy and loyal employees.

Race to the next chapter.

Chapter 8

CorYoga is a Tool

What do the following have in common: baseball, hockey, yoga, tennis, golf, chiropractic?

Answer: TWIST!!

Several years ago, I took a group of students on a yoga retreat to Tensing Pen in Negril, Jamaica. We had a great time. But while I was there, I decided to visit a local yoga studio in town in hopes of making friends. Since I was a yoga teacher there on a retreat, I thought we would have things in common and could share some ideas, and I could refer Canadian yoga students who are coming to Jamaica to go to this studio. While I was talking with the director or owner of the studio, she asked me what kind of yoga I teach. I told her I teach CorYoga, my own brand. She asked, "What is CorYoga?"

I told her, at which point she very boastfully told me that she teaches Ashtanga yoga, the best kind, and that no other kind compares with her style. I was just about to ask her what Ashtanga yoga was, but she didn't even give me the chance to ask the question; she just walked away slowly and angelically, as if she were floating on air. She walked away, leaving me with the impression that she wanted me to know that she was better than me. I did not make friends that day.

So what is it with some yoga teachers thinking and behaving like they are better than everybody else? Why do they often walk so slowly, like they have a special connection to the Devine that no one else has? What's up with that? We yoga people are supposed to be peaceful practicing people, yet we often display big egos and an "I am better than thou" attitude. When you take a look, you will find that this same attitude and behavior is a major source of war and fighting on this planet. So what's up with that? And what's the meaning of *better*?

Consider this: at one time in our history not too long ago, if you were a person of my colour, your life was worth almost nothing. Your worth would be less than a dog. And today, the most powerful man on this planet is a man of my colour. So, what's the meaning of *better*?

Who is better than who, and who says so? Who makes the rules? No human is better than another, and no style of yoga is better than another; they are just slightly different and serve slightly different purposes.

There is one thing that we need to understand, and that is: YOGA IS A TOOL!

It's a fantastic, multipurpose tool. Too many of us are making too much out of what it is. It's a great tool for golfers; it's a fantastic tool for healing low back pain; it's a great tool that we can use to get closer to that which we call the Devine, or God, or the Universe. Want some more? Yoga is a tool that we can use to help relieve depression.

Erin's Story

Several years ago while I was teaching yoga, I noticed a young girl who kept coming to class regularly and consistently. I wondered why this young, teenage girl kept coming to class. Shouldn't she be outside playing ball and making fun of boys? So one day I asked her why she was so dedicated to my yoga class. She told me she had chronic anxiety and depression, and my style of yoga was the only thing that helped her to feel better. That threw me for a mind spin. I couldn't figure out the connection. I figured CorYoga was on one hand and depression on the other hand—no connection! So one day I was training a private client who happened to be a Physiotherapist. I told her about this young girl being so dedicated to my CorYoga class and that she had told me that my CorYoga was the only thing that helped with her depression. I also told her that it made no sense to me and I didn't see any connection. So she said to me, "Lee, that's easy." I said, "Enlighten me." She then told me that depression is a chemical imbalance and, in yoga, when you make her bend and twist, you cause her to massage her internal organs, which causes them to secrete the proper quantity of hormones back into her blood and bring her body chemistry back into balance, which eases her depression. And bing! The light bulb went on, and the connection was made—I see it, I understand it, and it makes sense!

Yoga is a tool that can be used for many things, including easing depression. Subsequently, Erin went on to take my CorYoga teacher training program. I have certified her, and today she is a certified CorYoga teacher. If we could just stop using yoga to make us look like we are better than others and start using it as the great tool that it can be used for, we would all be much better off, living a peaceful and harmonious life.

Of all the tools that I have come across for healing back pain, the absolutely best one, without the shadow of a doubt, is yoga. Nothing else compares; yoga is the absolute best tool for healing back pain.

Why? Because yoga twisting poses adjust all the bones in your back; plus, yoga stretches the muscles, ligaments, and tendons of your back.

It's a tool for golfers:

Many golfers experience injuries from the following areas: hands, wrists, forearms, elbows, shoulders, hips, and knees. However, one of the most common injuries that a golfer endures is low back pain.

Here is why: during the off-season, many golfers tend to not do anything to condition their body. I figure that if you were to go out and tell some typical male golfer that he should do yoga, the first thing that he would probably do is kick you in the shin; then he would probably punch you in the face. Then, when you fall to the ground, he would spit in your face, kick you again in the ribs, and then he would take his golf club and beat you over your head. You see, it's difficult to get such athletes to do something like yoga, even though yoga is the best thing that a golfer can use to condition his or her body. And then, at the start of the golf season, without having conditioned the body over the off-season, he goes out, swings, and there goes the back.

If you tell a female golfer to do yoga to improve her game, no problem, she will do it. Try telling a male golfer, and you are in trouble. No way is he going to do it!! Tell him to spend $1000.00 on the newest golf club, and no problem!! Done!! Tell him to do some yoga, which costs him very little, and that it will alleviate his back pain. Forget it!! Here is the interesting thing. If you are experiencing low back pain, and you are in bed and can't move, it doesn't matter how expensive your golf club is; it doesn't matter how good your golf club is—you are not playing golf that day. At this point, your golf club is no good to you, and you are no good to your family or friends.

So, let's look at the other side of the equation. What if the golfer would take some time and do golfer's CorYoga? The first thing that would happen is he would experience improved core strength, balance, focus, and concentration, and, most importantly, he would experience improved flexibility. That means that when he swings his expensive golf club, his back would be loose enough that he wouldn't pull his muscles and hurt his back. His spine would be decompressed so that he would not compress his spine and herniate his disc. And, most importantly, his body would do what his golf pro is trying to make him do, which would result in an improved golf game.

Doesn't that make sense to you?

Does to me!!

As a golfer, you do one single movement. You swing a golf club. Now, I don't mean to simplify, minimize, criticize, or down play your sport. But while performing your sport, you don't run, jump, or shoot a ball; you don't jump and spike a ball, and you don't throw the ball with your hands. You swing a golf club. The action is complex; it requires precision, concentration, and a great deal of skills. But at the end of the day, you really do only one body movement—you swing a golf club. In CorYoga, we do this very same body movement but with variations. We call this action a twist, and there are many variations on this twist. Because of the many variations, a golfer can use this as a sport specific activity to help enhance their game. See fig. 1 below.

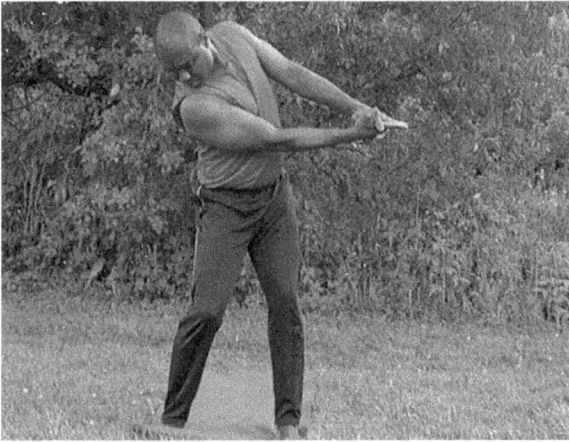

Fig. 1

For your free colour version of this photo, go to www.backcareworld.com.

Now, I know that this is not a proper gold stance, but then again this is not a lesson in golf. This is a CorYoga posture. But here is what this posture and golf has in common: they both require the upper body to rotate, coil, and uncoil. If you should do this posture over and over again in a yoga studio, guess what? Your body will get used to this motion, and then when you go out there on the course, your body will say, "Yup, I know this motion;

I have done it many times," so you will have less of a chance of hurting yourself when you swing a golf club. But whether you believe me or not, that doesn't make this posture useless to you. It is still very useful to you as a golfer. So, do it!!!

CorYoga makes your body loose, supple, flexible, and strong.

Subsequently, I have developed an app for golfers called *Golfers' CorYoga*. This app contains short, manageable videos that a golfer can do right on the golf course while playing the game. In fact, the app is designed to be used while playing the game.

I have walked along the road and have seen people walking with a cane or some kind of support, and it would look like their spine was completely rigid, and they were in a bent over position. Have you ever noticed people like that walking on the road?

More than once, I have seen old men walking with their heads bent forward so much that, from behind, you couldn't tell that they even have a head. Their heads would be completely not visible from behind.

I often asked myself what would happen if people would just do three rounds of sun salutations and a spinal twist just once per day. What would be the result of that? I'll tell you what that would do.

For sure, the spine would become more flexible, as the muscles of the back would become looser and more flexible. The spine would become decompressed on a regular basis, thereby becoming an antidote for spinal shrinkage. This means the person would not get shorter as the years go by. There would be less spinal disc bulging and less back pain for sure. The spine would maintain or increase its mobility. Because spinal disc compression and disc bulging can result in other complications such as sciatica or sexual dysfunction, or a host of other conditions, many, if not all, of these conditions would be avoided. This would result in improving spinal health, as well as your overall health, and the quality of your life would be greatly enhanced. And that would start by simply doing 2 or 3 rounds of sun salutations and spinal twists.

For your free video of sun salutation and spinal twist, go to www.backcareworld.com.

The best way to keep the spine in proper alignment is to do a type of yoga posture called spinal twist.

Now, some doctors will tell you to never twist your spine. I don't know why, but I have heard many people say that. But I would like you to consider this: isn't this twisting motion the basis of the chiropractic principles? Isn't that twisting motion what they do to you when they adjust you? That's what they did to me for 27 years as a chiropractic patient. But maybe we should take a look at what a spinal twist is.

What is a spinal twist?

See the section on Spinal Twist in Chapter 6.

When you are standing upright, the orientation of your shoulders is on the same plane as the orientation of your hips. When the orientation of your shoulders moves away from the plane of the orientation of your hips, starting to approach 90 degrees opposite from your hips, that becomes a spinal twist. The closer your hips and shoulders are in approaching 90 degrees to each other, the better your twist is.

Some people's spinal twists are fantastic, while others are lousy (like mine). But, no problem, I have other strengths as a yoga teacher.

I remember this one time when a young man came to a CorYoga class that I was teaching. It was his first ever yoga class. The moment I started to do the sitting spinal twist, he not only did the twist perfectly, he went straight into a full pretzel. In that moment, I wanted to go straight over to him and beat him up. Why? Because for as long as I can remember, I have been trying to do a pretzel, and I have never been able to accomplish it. And now, here comes this new whipper snapper person, moving effortlessly into a perfect pretzel, just like that. He probably doesn't even know how to spell the word yoga (like me when I started). Anyway, that is great for him. Some people's bodies are just not meant to rotate or move that way, and I am just one of those people—I accept that; I can live with that; and I am moving on.

So, with all this talk about spinal twists and perfect pretzels, what's the benefits of all this, and what does it have to do with back pain?

Well, first of all, the first and most important function of the spinal twist is to adjust and realign the back and spine. This is the foundation of the Chiropractic principle. The concept is to realign the spine on a regular basis so to alleviate stress off the spinal nerve and alleviate back pain. When the body is in proper alignment in equilibrium, it functions much better and thereby facilitates self-healing and maintains proper health.

Secondly, the spinal twist and pretzel aids in digestion and elimination. When you do a spinal twist, you massage and squeeze your internal organs. The massaging and squeezing forces material through, thereby aiding with elimination. The squeezing also forces out stale blood and brings in fresh blood, which brings in fresh oxygen and nutrients that nourish your internal organs, and thereby makes them function better.

Makes sense?

Good!!

In fact, the spinal twist not only adjusts the spine and brings it back into balance, it also stretches and strengthens the muscles along the spine, keeping the spine loose, supple, and strong on a regular basis. When these muscles are loose and supple, they stop pulling on the spine and reduce tension and pain, if not eliminating pain altogether.

The spinal twist is one of the most useful and functional yoga postures there is.

Why?

Because the spinal twist serves the golfers, the hockey players, and the baseball players, and a myriad of other people who play sports. These are just the obvious ones.

So, all this commotion about not twisting your body is hog wash. Here is what I believe you should not do. Don't lift heavy objects and twist without moving your legs. When you lift heavy objects, you tend to compress your spine; then, when you turn without moving your legs, you can cause a disc to move out of place and press on spinal nerves, causing pain. If you are going to lift an object, bend your knees, pick it up, stand upright, move your legs, and turn your entire body, not just your upper body.

While a Chiropractor usually adjusts a specific part of the spine, a CorYoga twist will affect the entire spine because we do many variations of the spinal twist.

See the section on Spinal Twist in Chapter 6.

Sun Salutation and spinal twist works in keeping the spine healthy. It works, and I am the living example of that.

So, why won't we do it? I'll tell you why we won't do it—because it works!!

Have you noticed that we won't do many simple things that are good for us, but we are so eager to do the things that are not good for us? Want a few examples? Many people smoke when we have much proof that smoking kills the human body. Many of us drink excessively when we know psoriasis of the liver kills. If you think about it, I am sure you can think of more examples, both from a personal level to a professional level, and to the community level, all the way up to the federal government level where things make sense and are good for the majority of the community; we won't do it, but things that makes no sense for the community, that's what they will do. Why is that? Why don't you do whatever it takes to maintain good spinal health? Know what the funniest and craziest thing is? We spend so many hours each and every day doing things that will benefit other people, but we won't take 20 minutes each day to do something to maintain the health of our spine. Want to hear something even crazier? When we do some physical exercise, such as sun salutation and spinal twist, only we ourselves get the benefits—not our boss or our spouse or anybody else. We alone, except for our offspring, get all the benefits from the exercise.

And we are happy sacrificing ourselves by doing good things for others when we won't do the same for ourselves. That's not bad or good; it just is. And you know what that tells me? We innately know that we are all here on this planet not for ourselves but for others. We are here to help other people to get better. That's why we have children. When we have children, we dedicate our entire lives to them. We are for others. Everything we do is for somebody else. We work for somebody else. We have children for somebody else (the children). My grandmother and my aunt gave of their time and energy to save me so that I may give of my time, knowledge, and energy to serve, help, and save you; and you will give of your time, energy, and knowledge to save and help others—and the endless circle continues. And the sooner we understand and work with this, the easier it will be for us to live a peaceful and harmonious life.

Race to chapter 9 to learn how to stay young.

Chapter 9

Anti-Aging CorYoga

Reincarnation is for real! If you think that you are the same person who existed 7 year ago, you would not be correct. Every single day, you have body cells that are dying and new cells that are being born. Scientists have determined that every seven years, your entire body has completely replaced its old cells with all new ones. Therefore, every seven years you become a new person. That's actually a good thing! That means that starting right now, you can start to take steps to ensure that when new cells are being born, they are born as healthy as possible. Then, all you have to do is just do whatever it takes to have them remain healthy and young as possible, thereby retarding the aging process.

How do you like that?

So, what's one step that we can take to make this happen? One thing that we can do to help with this process is that we can feed ourselves as best we can. Therefore, eat the freshest organic fruits and vegetables. The next thing that we can do is get lots of good quality sleep. That means going to bed between 10:30 and 11:30 p.m.

Good quality food will supply the nutrients so that when your body repairs itself, it will repair itself to the youngest you possible. Does that make sense to you?

It doesn't matter; do it anyway!!

OK, so that's one way to retard the aging process.

Let's look at another way that we can retard the aging process but, before we do, let's consider this scenario: it's early evening; the sun has just gone down, and it's just starting to turn dark. It is somewhere between light and dark, and the city lights are just starting to come on (if you are living in a city).

You are walking down the street. Coming towards you are two individuals. One of the individuals is on your right hand side and the other on your left hand side. You cannot make out any details of these individuals, but you can tell that the one on your right hand side is walking slowly and gingerly with a cane, and he is looking downward with shoulders slumped forward and downward.

Do you have that picture?

Good!!

On your left hand side, the person is walking briskly, without a cane, with head held high, and shoulders up and backwards.

Got that picture?

Excellent!

Now, if you had to give an answer, which one would you categorize as the older person? If you are like most people, you would say the one on your right.

Right?

Why?

Because that person displays characteristics of an older person, walking slowly, with a cane, head held low, with shoulders slumped forward and downward. People who display such characteristics, we judge them and categorize them as old.

But what if that person on your right (the one appearing old) is actually a 20-year-old person who is experiencing severe back pain, and the one on your left is actually an 85-year-old person who exercises and does yoga regularly?

The purpose of this scenario is to illustrate to you that we judge people as old based on their behavior, as well as the way they look. If you walk hunched over, we judge you as old. In fact, the more hunched over you walk, the older we say you are. If you walk vertically upright, with head up, chest up, shoulders up and backwards, we say you are young. Right? Right!!

So, how does long term sitting and working in an office cause you to age, and how can we slow down or reverse that process?

When you sit for a long time in your office, and you neglect to stretch your body, the muscles in the front of your hips (your hip flexors) get tight and shortened over time. If this continues, the tight muscles pull your bottom from underneath your spine and causes you to be hunched over at the hips. The more this continues, the tighter they become; the more hunched over you become, the older you become or appear to be.

How can we reverse this?

Simple—get on a regular program of stretching out your hip flexors. Follow the pictures below. This posture is what we call anti-aging posture, because it keeps your hip flexors loose and supple, and stops you from walking hunched over like an old person.

Follow the posture below; this is a solution to tighten hip flexor muscles.

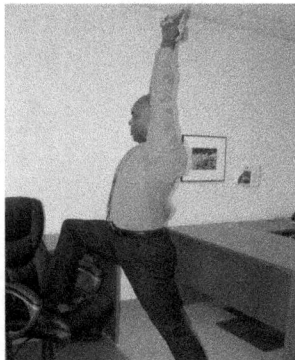

Fig. 1

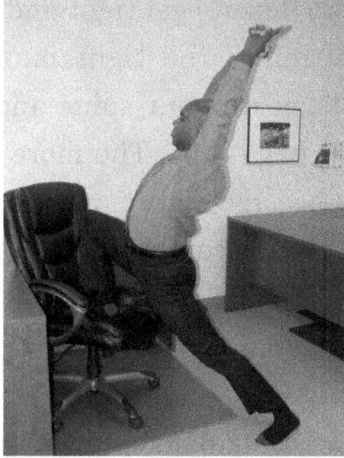

Fig. 2

For your free colour version of these photos, go to
www.backcareworld.com.

Anti-Aging Benefits of Yoga

Yoga can slow the aging process by improving some
key factors of physical health that are related to aging.

Here are 5 of them:

Flexibility:

Spinal flexibility is about quality of life and not just
comfort.

Regular CorYoga practice creates spinal flexibility, which creates space between the vertebrae, which helps lengthen the spine, in turn improving nerve conduction to all the organs which helps keep you young.

This can be summed up in one phrase: when the wind comes, the flexible tree will bend, but the rigid tree will break. So, keep the spine flexible and retard the aging process.

Blood glucose and insulin:

People tend to develop abdominal obesity with normal aging. Abdominal obesity has a link to type 2 diabetes. CorYoga has a very positive effect on that. But allow me to tell you my story.

About 8 years ago, my mother and her husband developed type 2 diabetes and had to start taking insulin injections. They lived in Hamilton, Ontario, about a 1 hour drive from where I live and teach CorYoga in Toronto. I encouraged them to come to take CorYoga with me. After a while, they decided to come and take CorYoga with me on Saturday mornings. I remember being so very happy to see my mom in my class, sweating with the rest of my students. I was so very proud of her and her husband. After about 4 Saturday classes in a row, the amount of insulin that they had to take dropped drastically. And then they stopped coming.

Bummer!! I was heartbroken. I tried to get my mom to move her body in other ways, but she was not interested. In March 2015, I buried my mother. She died of complications from type 2 diabetes. Here is the thing: I am the founder of CorYoga, and I have been teaching it for about 25 years. My father has diabetes, but he is still alive and doing well. My mother's mother (my grandmother) has diabetes. I don't have any diabetes, but I do get my blood sugar tested regularly. So, what if my mother didn't stop and had continued coming to CorYoga class with me?

Where would she be today? I don't know, but probably not six feet under. Anyway, you draw your own conclusion. All I know is that I am very convinced that if she had continued taking CorYoga with me, she would still be alive today.

Balance:

Balance actually means being in equilibrium.

A major component of most yoga posture is balance. For example, think of the tree pose, triangle pose and, of course, don't forget the warrior pose. The warrior pose, especially the warrior 1, is anti-aging in more ways than one. First of all, warrior 1 retards the aging process by cultivating balance. Both the brain and the body is involved in balance, and when one or both faculties are not used, they will diminish. Secondly, when you sit for a long period of time, your hip flexors will get tighter. Over time, those tight hip flexors will pull your bottom from under your spine and cause you to walk bending forward. People who walk bent forward, we categorize as old. But when you practice warrior 1 posture, it stretches out the hip flexors and thus keeps you walking upright and, therefore, we say you are young.

Life is a balancing act. The universe is balanced, and it will remain that way no matter what we say, do, or think.

Here are a few examples from my experience:

I have a website called www.c2cfit.com. It is a website that challenges everyone to exercise their way around the world without leaving home. I have many children on the site taking part in the challenge. I had

Google Ads on the site so that if members clicked the ads, Google would pay me money, if it accumulated to $100.00 US or more. After about 3 months of watching and waiting, it finally accumulated to just over $100.00. I had been anxious to get that check from Google because it was the fruits of my labor, and it would prove to me that Google Ads really works. It was then that I received an email from Google saying that they had disabled my account because I have illegal clicks. I was completely heartbroken because, honestly, it wasn't me who illegally clicked the ads, if there were illegal clicks. I suspected that it was one of the kids on the site who illegally clicked the ads, because that's what kids do (things that they aren't supposed to do). If Google had checked the IP address connected to the illegal clicks, they would have realized that it wasn't me because, honestly, it wasn't me who illegally clicked the ads. I sent Google an email, but they have never replied. The only thing I could do was feel bad about it, forget it, and move along with my broken heart. About 2 months after that, it was in the winter, and I was walking along one of the narrow walkways through the low rise complex of my condominium, going to work. I looked ahead, and coming towards me was a young man in his 40s and a little girl, maybe around 7 years old. As they walked past me, I said, "Hi," and they replied and walked by.

About 4 steps away from where we passed each other, I saw something unusual on the ground. I stopped and picked it up. It was a brand new $100.00 US bill. I quickly turned around to give it to the man who had just passed me, as I thought that he had dropped it, even though I didn't see him drop it. But both he and the little girl had completely disappeared. I looked around to see if I could find him, but there wasn't a trace of them. So, I thought, "Umm, it's not a life or death situation." So I put it in my pocket and, as I walked away, I thought to myself, "Could this be the $100.00 US that Google owed me and refused to pay me?" I thought, "Umm, the universe is balanced and will remain that way, regardless of what we say, do, or think."

The second example occurred in July of 2011. I went into the subway at Wellesley and Yonge, coming back uptown from teaching a CorYoga class. I reached into my pocket and pulled out a token to pay but, as my hand came out of my pocket with the token, it fell out of my hand and on to the floor. I looked around to pick up the token but it had completely disappeared. It was as if the token had fallen into a black hole. It was nowhere to be found. I thought, "It's not a life and death situation. It will come back to me. I have another token in my pocket, so I will just use another one and move along as I have another class uptown to teach in 45 minutes." So, that is precisely what I did—paid another token and went along.

Two weeks later, I was sitting at Starbucks, Yonge and Avondale, outside on the patio writing this very book that you are reading now. I was sitting out on the patio writing when this lady got up from another table and started walking towards the stop light. As she walked by me, I heard something fall on the ground. I looked around to see what it was. About two seconds later, I saw the token on the ground that she had dropped. I yelled at her, "Excuse me, hey lady, hello," but by that time she was in the middle of the intersection, crossing the street. I picked up the token and started walking after her when the lights changed. I thought, "Umm, it's not a life or death situation." I went back to sitting at my table and continued writing this book. Then I thought, "Could this be the token that I had lost in the subway 2 weeks ago? I thought, "Umm! The universe is balanced and will remain so, regardless of what we say, do, or think.

Whatever you do, strive to maintain balance. Do you want a good relationship? It's about balance. In yoga, there are a number of things that will affect your balance, some of which are strength of opposing muscle groups, orientation of your head, brightness of the environment, and where you are looking (focus), and more. You will find that in actual relationships, these same elements will determine the strength and stability of your relationship. If one partner pushes or pulls too much, that will bring the relationship out of equilibrium, and the relationship won't last. Without balance, a relationship will die. Balance is anti-aging in more ways than one.

Energy:

It was June of 2011, and I was in a hot room teaching a hot CorYoga class. I remember going over and adjusting a student's back and then just rubbing it after the adjustment. Then I moved on to helping other students. At the end of class, she came up to me and asked, "Lee, do you do Reiki?" I answered, "No, why do you ask?" She said, "Today, I came to class with back pain and, after you touched my back, the pain completely went away."

The question is this: was it the physical CorYoga posture that healed her, or was it energy from me through my hands?

I don't know!

Did I touch her with the intention to heal her?

Are you kidding? I had no idea she had back pain until she spoke to me after class!

Could I do this again? I have no idea, not a clue!

Do I believe in all this energy work?

Absolutely!!

I believe that we are walking around thinking that we are physical beings, but the fact is that we are more energy beings than physical beings— quantum physics tells us that. If you accept the notion that we are energy beings, and since physics tells us that energy can neither be created nor destroyed, then it makes logical sense that we cannot die; we can only change from one form to another. Some people had learned how to use their energy, while some people had not learned that yet. Some people are consciously aware that they are using their *chi* or *internal energy* for destructive or beneficial purposes, and some are not aware (like I was not aware that I was using my energy to heal her back when I adjusted Mariam).

Everything is energy, and energy is everything.

Can you think of any examples from your life to exemplify the fact that the universe is balanced?

Assignment: Please go to my website at www.back careworld.com and submit it there.

Chapter 10

The Program

Now you know the major causes of back pain, the financial cost of treating back pain, and that the solution is yoga. So, what kind of yoga program would be most suitable for treating and alleviating back pain, especially when you are in your office?

The goal of this program is to do two things: to decompress the spine and also to stretch out the spine and the muscles of the spine.

Like Dr. McCall said, *"In order to have a healthy back and spine, you need to have a forward bend, side bend, tilt, backbend, and a twist in your stretching program, in order to keep your spinal discs supple and nourished."*

If there is only one thing that you could find time to do at work in order to alleviate back pain, it should be the *Standing Forward Bend.* Why?

See the fig 1a and 1b below.

Because it is the easiest, simplest, and most effective way to decompress your spine and stretch out tight and tired muscles.

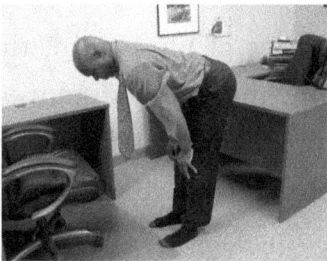 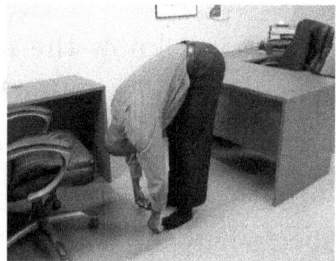

Fig. 1a   *Fig. 1b*

For your free colour version of these photos, go to
www.backcareworld.com.

Here is how it's done. Stand with your feet together. Bring your hands together and inhale. Reach your hands straight up into the air. This serves to lengthen your spine. Then, as you exhale, sweep your arms out to the side and come to a forward fold, just like in the figure above.

The magic of this posture comes when you inhale and come up, and exhale and go down into the posture. It gives life to the posture by adding movement and breath. It also allows you to go deeper into the posture, thus getting you a fuller, deeper stretch. It also prevents injury to your body.

One more big advantage happens when you do this:

When you exhale while going into a posture, something happens to your muscles, and this feeling translates into your entire body. We call this feeling *relaxation.* So, each and every time that you exhale and go into the posture, you are relaxing your entire body with every breath. This is more beneficial than going into a posture and holding it statically until it's time to move to the next posture.

This posture is extremely beneficial, especially if you cross your legs while doing this standing forward bend. You can see this entire series of posture on my website, www.backcareworld.com.

Standing Back Bend

In order to counteract the bending position of the sitting forward bend, you should then do a standing back bend which is the next posture that I recommend in this program. And this is another one of those postures that you can use as a camouflage to what you are actually doing. So, stand with your legs approximately shoulder width apart, and bring your hands to your buttocks. Then, bend backwards and look up to the ceiling as if you are checking something on the ceiling. The key thing to remember when doing this posture is to relax your butt muscles. The benefit of this posture is that it stretches the muscles of the lumbar spine and, as well, it opens the lower back vertebrae. Once again, you want to add the dynamic motion of inhaling and coming up, and exhaling and going backwards into the posture.

And if someone walks in on you, all you have to do is pretend you are checking for something on the ceiling. Cool? Cool!

Here is what it looks like:

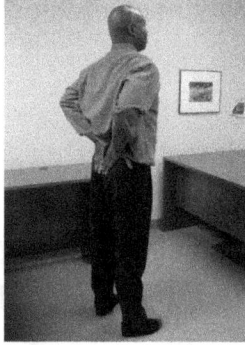

Fig. 2a

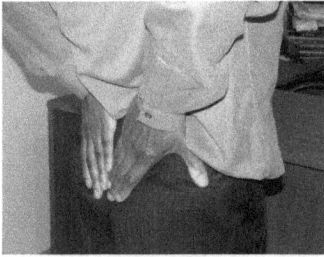

Fig. 2b

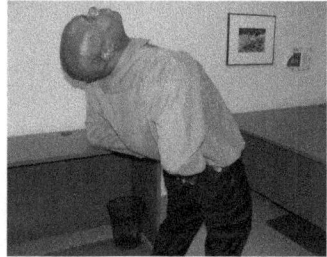

Fig. 2c

For your free colour version of these photos, go to
www.backcareworld.com.

Standing Side Tilt

There is a muscle at the side of your body that is directly responsible for back pain. This muscle is called the quadratus lumborum. When this muscle gets tight, it pulls on the vertebrae and causes your spine to compress to the side, which causes your spinal disc to bulge out, putting pressure on the spinal nerve, which causes pain. The way to stretch out this muscle is to do a standing side tilt.

Stand with both feet together. Send your right arm up into the sky and reach up toward the sky. As you exhale, tilt to your left side. Once again, inhale and come up, and exhale and tilt to your left. Repeat about 6 times and switch.

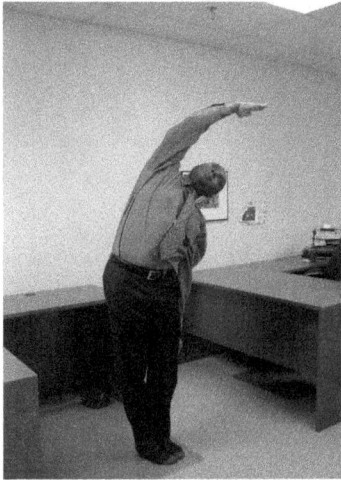

Fig. 3a

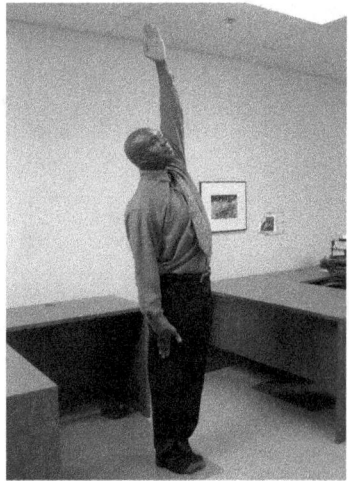

Fig. 3b

For your free colour version of these photos, go to
www.backcareworld.com.

No Pain, Your Gain

Standing Spinal Twist

If you have time (and you should make time) to do a second series of posture, let it be the *standing spinal twist* or the *sitting spinal twist*.

If you choose to do the standing spinal twist, this would be good as it gives you a chance to stand instead of sit. A second benefit is that it twists and realigns the spine.

From a standing position, place your right leg on top of your chair. Place your left hand on your right leg and your right hand on your left butt cheek. Twist and turn to your right side while using your left hand to pull yourself a little further to the right. Inhale and come around facing front again, and then exhale and twist turn to your right. Repeat and then switch sides.

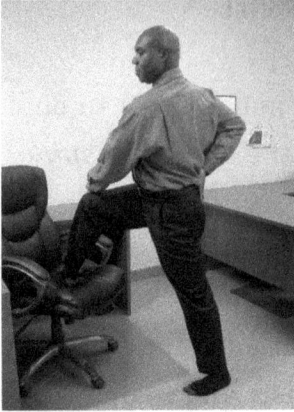

Fig. 4a

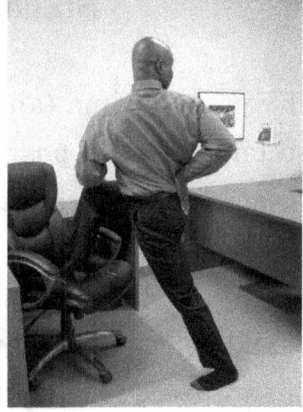

Fig. 4b

For your free colour version of these photos, go to
www.backcareworld.com.

Standing Prayer Twist

For this posture, you are going to place your left leg
flat on your chair, and make sure that your foot is firmly
planted on the chair. Then, take your right elbow to the
outside of your left leg. Turn your right palm on top of
your left palm and push into the outside edge of your left
leg, twisting to the left side. Then, inhale and come
around and, as you exhale, twist and turn to your left
side. Repeat, and then switch legs. One benefit of this
posture is that it twists and realigns the back and spine.
As well, it aids in digestion and elimination.

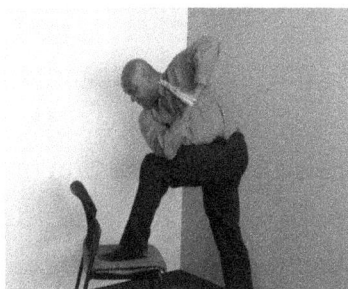

Fig. 5a

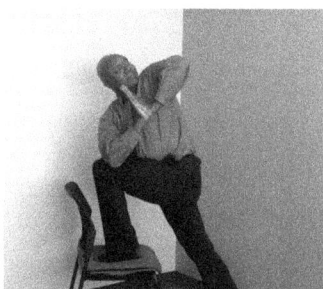

Fig. 5b

For your free colour version of these photos, go to
www.backcareworld.com.

The next series of posture that I highly recommend
is the *stand reach and hold.*

Stand Reach and Hold

If you speak with any reputable physiotherapist,
they will tell you that tight hamstrings will usually lead
to low back pain. I don't know why, but anyone with
tight hamstrings usually ends up experiencing back
pain. So, what can one do about tight hamstrings? First,
place your right leg on top of your chair, and point your
toes toward your head. Keep your leg fairly straight
without locking the knee joint. Then, place your hands
on your right leg and, as you exhale, slide them down
toward your foot and bring your head down towards

your knee. As you do that, try to point your toes up towards your head. This will give you a stronger, heightened awareness in the back of your legs (the hamstrings). Once again, include the dynamic motion by inhaling and coming up, and exhaling and sliding down. The benefit of this posture is that it stretches out the back of your leg, the hamstring, and it also stretches out your lower back, middle back, and upper back.

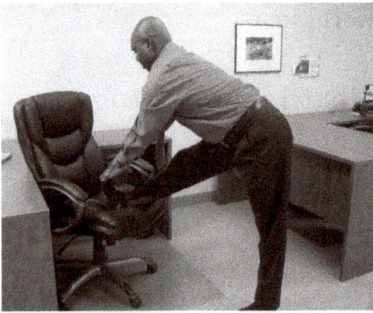 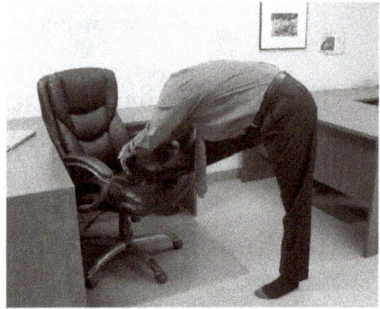

Fig. 6a   *Fig. 6b*

For your free colour version of these photos, go to www.backcareworld.com.

Standing Back Stretch (on back of chair)

As you can see from the photo below, this posture is very easy and simple to do, yet it is highly effective in stretching out the shoulders, the entire back and spine, the gluteus, and hamstring. This is a stretch that everyone should do daily in the office. And again, this is another one of those poses that you can do and pretend that you are doing something else. So, turn the back of your chair so that it is facing you, and hold on to the top of the chair back. Then, open your legs to approximately shoulder width apart. Drop your head in between your shoulders and allow your body to fall down towards the floor. Inhale and come up, and exhale and go down. Repeat as many times as you feel necessary. If someone walks in on you, just pretend that you are looking for a pen that you dropped on the floor; so, before you start, remember to put a pen on the floor in front of you.

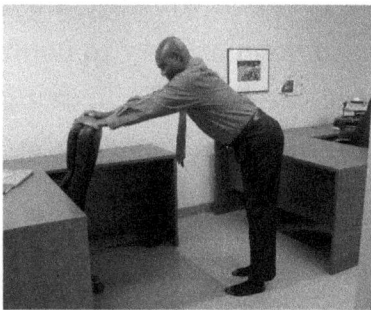
Fig. 7a

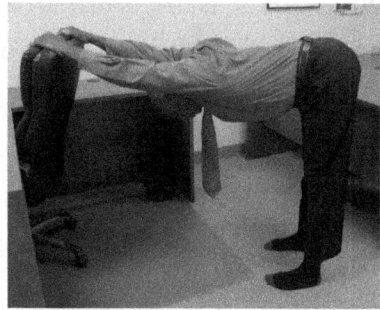
Fig. 7b

For your free colour version of these photos, go to
www.backcareworld.com.

Sitting Forward Bend

The next series of posture, which is the *sitting forward bend*, is really cool. Since you are going to be doing this stretch in your office, I recommend you hold a pen in your hand while doing this. That way if someone walks into your office while you are sitting and bending forward, you can just say, "Oh, there it is," and come back up to a sitting position with your pen in your hand. That way, they would just think you were bending over to pick up your pen from the floor.

How?

Sit at the edge of your chair with your legs apart and wide open. Bring your arms in between your legs and, as you exhale, come to a forward bend and try to point the crown of your head towards the floor. Then, bring your hands to your thigh and inhale while coming up, and exhale while going down. Repeat as many times as you feel you need to.

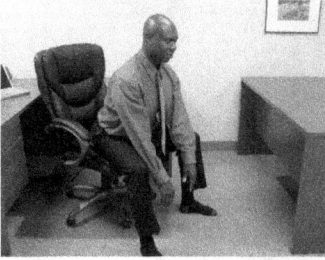

Fig. 8a

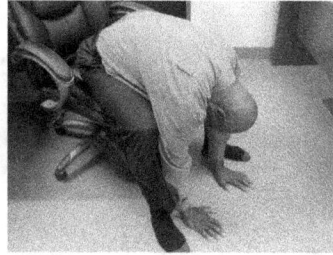

Fig. 8b

For your free colour version of these photos, go to www.backcareworld.com.

Sitting Head to Toes Stretch

Since you were just standing up, I will get you to sit down again. So, the next posture is the *sitting head to toe stretch*. The benefit of this posture is that it stretches the muscles of the middle back, lower back, and, most importantly, the hips. As you have been sitting for a while, most people's hips tend to get tight and painful. Well, this is one posture that stretches the hips. So, sit at the front edge of your chair, raise your left leg, and cross your right leg above your knee. Place your left arm on your left leg and inhale; as you exhale, you will press down on your leg while folding forward and bringing your head toward your leg. Repeat three times and switch legs.

This is what it looks like:

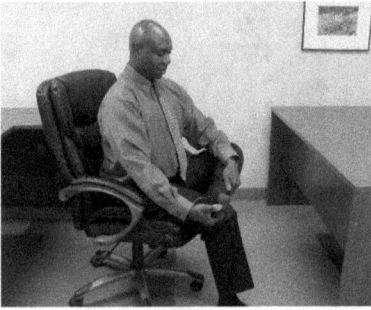 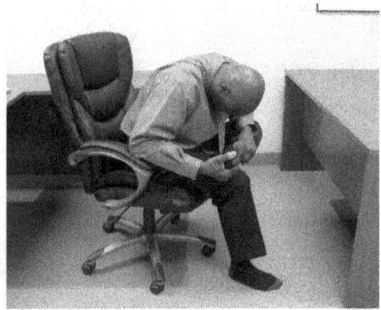

Fig. 9a   *Fig. 9b*

For your free colour version of these photos, go to

www.backcareworld.com.

Sit Reach and Hold

Here is an all-in-one posture. This sit reach and hold posture stretches almost all of the muscles in the back of your body, from your calves to your hamstrings, to your glutei, lower back, middle back, upper back, shoulders, and neck.

Sit on the floor with your legs straight. Bring your hands together. Inhale and reach your arms up towards the sky and, as you exhale, reach your arms forward towards your toes. When you reach up before you fold forwards, this serves to lengthen the spine first so you don't crunch your spine as you fold forward. It doesn't matter if you can touch your toes or not; it only matters that you feel a stretch and breathe long, deep fluidic breaths. Once again, add life to the posture by inhaling and coming up, and by exhaling and going down. Repeat.

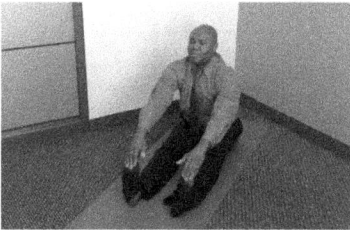 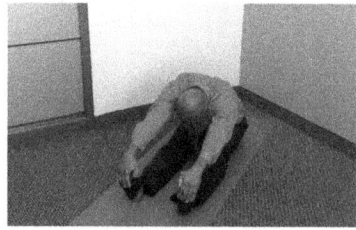

Fig. 10a　　　　　　　　*Fig. 10b*

For your free colour version of these photos, go to www.backcareworld.com.

Lying Down

Of all the amazing things that you can do in the middle of the work day to alleviate back pain, there is nothing you can do that is better than lying down flat on your back.

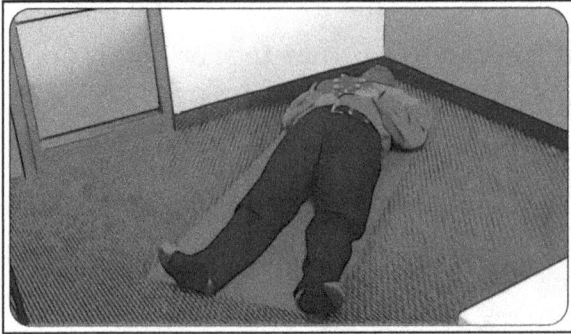

Fig. 11

There is nothing like it. It reduces the downward pull of gravity on your spinal disc and, therefore, alleviates the spinal compression caused by long term sitting or standing. It facilitates easy blood flow to your head, which increases fresh oxygen and nutrients and allows you to think much clearer and be more reasonable when you come back to a standing or sitting position.

If there is only one thing that you can do to alleviate back pain, let it be lying down flat on your back. Everyone, in every company, should lie down flat on their back at least once (better yet twice) per day at work. It is a civilized thing to do.

Dweet!! (This is Jamaican for *Do It*!)

Your final assignment:

If you are an executive or are in management at any company, try this: before you go into any meeting or negotiation, just pick one or two of the stretches that I mentioned above and do them. Then, immediately lie down flat on your back for about 15 minutes, and then get up and go to your meeting. Then, stay aware of how you feel or how you perform during the meeting. This will rest your tired back, refresh you, rejuvenate you, make you think clearer, and better prepare you for your meeting or negotiation. And this could help your company to improve productivity and profitability.

This exercise program that I just gave you above is a shortened down version of a more extended video program that I have for you at my website. Go there now, purchase your membership, and start doing the video exercises. Start living the way you deserve to live, with no pain and more gain.

About the Author

For 27 years, Lee has lived with severe low back pain. But now he has absolutely no back pain. He has had almost every treatment that one can think of for low back pain. None of these treatments were able to help him eliminate his back pain. So, Lee developed a style of yoga which he used to heal himself, as well as many of his students (See testimonials in this book.) Today, Lee is presenting his OYO Back Care program to offices of companies that are interested in helping their employees to find ways to de-stress at their desks, alleviate back pain, and improve productivity and profitability. Lee has successfully licensed his online OYO Back Care Program to the Ontario Hospital Association and the Ministry of Municipal Affairs and Housing, among others.

For a list of some of Lee's recent clients, please see the acknowledgement section in this book.

Lee is also a certified Life Coach and a certified Mastermind Facilitator. He is available for Speaking, Training, Mastermind, Life Coaching and Workshop.

If you are interested in having Lee come to your company to work with your team on back care for office workers, please contact him at:

Lee Downer
Email: lee@backcareworld.com
Website: www.backcareworld.com
Phone: (416)209-9743

Work Cited

"Aching backs impact cost, disability." American
Academy of Orthopaedic Surgeons. American Academy
of Orthopaedic Surgeons, 2009. Web. 23 Jan. 2017.
<http://www.aaos.org/AAOSNow/2009/Jan/research/res
earch6/? ssopc=1>.

Ch. 3 page 7
Ch. 4. Page 5
Ch. 5 page 1
Ch. 6 page 1

Bohinski, Robert MD. "Herniated Lumbar Disc,"
Mayfield Brain and Spine. Mayfield Brain and Spine,
Apr. 2016. Web. 23 Jan. 2017. < http://www.
mayfieldclinic.com/PE-HLdisc.htm#.Vn4ovTZfnBp>.

Ch. 4 page 2

Research Findings. "Yoga for Healthy Lower Backs,"
N.P N.D. Web. 23 Jan. 2017. <
http://www.yogaforbacks.co.uk/research-findings/>.

Ch. 5 page 2

"Yoga: a cost-effective treatment for back pain sufferers?" Arthritis research UK. Arthritis research UK, 16 Aug. 2012. Web. 23 Jan. 2017. < http://www.arthritisresearchuk.org/news/press-releases/2012/august/yoga-a-cost-effective-treatment-fo r-back-pain-sufferers.aspx>.

Ch. 5 Page 5

"The science on lower back pain," CBC Player, CBC Radio-Canada, 15 Feb. 2016. Web. 23 Jan. 2016. < http://www.cbc.ca/player/play/2683730625>.

Ch. 6 Page 1

MCCALL, TIMOTHY M.D. "38 Health Benefits of Yoga," Yoga Journal, 28. Aug. 2007. Web. 23 Jan. 2017. < http://www.yogajournal.com/article/health/count-yoga-38-ways-yoga-keeps-fit/> .

Ch. 6 page 5

Merhar, Christina "Employee Retention - The Real Cost of Losing an Employee," Zane Benefits, 4 Feb. 2016. Web. 23 Jan. 2017 https://www.zanebenefits.com/blog/bid/312123/employe e-retention-the-real-cost-of-losing-an-employee.

Ch. 7 page 1

Webster, Victoria. "11 Most Surprising Famous People Who Loved To Nap," The Carousel. The Carousel. 8 Apr. 2016. Web. 23 Jan. 2017. < http://www.thecarousel.com/health/11-most-surprising-famous-people-who-loved-to-nap/>.

Ch. 7 Pages 5, 6

Guastini, Sherry. "5 Anti-Aging Benefits Of Yoga," Mindbodygreen. Mindbodygreen. 13 Jan. 2015. Web. 23 Jan. 2017. <http://www.mindbodygreen.com/0-16957/5-anti-aging-benefits-of-yoga.html>.

Ch. 9 pages 3, 4

www.ingramcontent.com/pod-product-compliance
Lightning Source LLC
Chambersburg PA
CBHW050652270326
41927CB00012B/2986

* 9 7 8 1 7 7 2 7 7 1 4 1 1 *